MW00487750

Enzymes:
Go With Your Gut

More Practical Guidelines
for Digestive Enzymes

———

Karen DeFelice

Many blessings
Karen DeFelice
www.enzymestuff.com

All rights reserved. No part of this publication may be reproduced in
any material form (including photocopying or storing it in any medium by
electronic means and whether or not transiently or incidentally to some other
use of this publication) without the written permission of
the copyright owner. The doing of an unauthorized act in relation
to a copyright work may result in both a civil claim for
damages and criminal prosecution.

Karen Leigh DeFelice is identified as author of this work in
accordance with the Copyright, Designs and Patents Act 1988.
Copyright Karen DeFelice 2006.

―――

Published by ThunderSnow Interactive
Printed and Bound Minnesota USA
ISBN 0-9725918-9-3

Other books by author:
Enzymes for Autism and other Neurological Conditions
The Practical Guide for Digestive Health and Better Behavior
ISBN 0-9725918-7-7

Enzymes for Digestive Health and Nutritional Wealth
The Practical Guide for Digestive Enzymes
ISBN 0-9725918-6-9

―――

Cover photo by Michael S. DeFelice
Cover designs by Karen DeFelice
Illustrations by Karen DeFelice,
Matthew DeFelice, and Michael S. DeFelice

Contents

LIST OF ILLUSTRATIONS

Acknowledgements

I would like to thank all the reviewers, especially the individuals doing the technical and scientific reviews, and those that contributed ideas, information, and direction ensuring the information was accurate to the best of our ability, and improving the quality of this work.

I especially want to thank the many, many volunteer individuals - everyday guys and gals - who worked with enzymes, researched on their own, and shared their views and findings. Sometimes the smallest detail can lead to fundamental discoveries and guidelines.

Extraordinary thanks to Tom Bohager and his team at Enzymedica and Theramedix for providing access to their technical resources and medical support network. They had the vision, integrity, and dedication to support education in enzyme therapy in a multitude of ways, often without compensation, forging ahead even when others lost interest. His team put into practice researching and developing specific enzymes for many health conditions. This has been a benefit and blessing to countless people as well as other organizations.

Thanks to David Thropp of Thropps Nutritionals for sharing his insight into certain matters of enzyme development that proved to be a key factor in finding solutions for certain families and individuals.

Special thanks go to Lisa Clark for countless hours committed to a calling that began in October 1998 when she coordinated the team and watched over the project to develop digestive enzymes for children with special needs. She kept this effort going, often quietly in the background, as it passed through its ups and down; maintaining the vision and faciliated it becoming reality even as others bowed out. Her friendship and support has been invaluable.

To my dear husband Dr. Michael DeFelice and my two wonderful sons for just being the profound blessings of my life. Especially for Mike's patience, support, guidance, and love all these years.

And thanks to our Great Lord God
through Whom all things are made possible.

Introduction

This book is a follow-up to my previous enzyme books, *Enzymes for Autism and other Neurological Conditions* and the variation *Enzymes for Digestive Health and Nutritional Wealth*. The first title, *Enzymes for Autism*, was intended to be a basic practical handbook to digestive enzymes and enzyme therapy for those with no background in this subject. The book quickly exceeded expectations. Many requests for a similar book for the general population flooded in leading to a mild variation, *Enzymes for Digestive Health*, coming out shortly afterwards. Either serves equally well as a great introduction to enzyme therapy since the core content is the same. In this book, I will refer to these titles jointly as *Enzymes for Autism/Digestive Health*.

Since the previous works, enzyme therapy has continued to advance and further discoveries and questions arose. Newer discoveries, more questions, special situations, and additional information became available. This book continues with content not covered in my previous books. In general, this book does not go into details already discussed in the other titles. However, some of the concepts previously covered are discussed from a different perspective, or explained in another way to help clarify the overall idea. References to the previous books are provided at particular points instead of repeating large amounts of detail should you want more information.

The chapters in this book focus on practical information supported with scientific references where available. Certain sections emphasize tips, tricks, and best practices to provide ideas and suggestions that may help you get better results with digestive enzymes if you are not currently seeing the improvements you hoped for. Guidelines for specific situations are based on what has worked for many people and provide the best chance for success. The information given is intended to serve as guidelines only which can easily be adapted to individual situations.

The last chapter is a troubleshooting guide containing common situations that may crop up once a person begins enzymes. Some are related to enzymes while others deal with general health. Suggestions for specific issues are meant to be 'best bet' ideas to help you streamline all the available alternatives. The goal is to simplify the myriad of choices available, focusing on simpler, practical, cost-effective yet efficient and effective options. It is not meant to be an all-inclusive list of everything that could possibly work.

There is again an extensive reference section. The 'Reference' section includes the references noted in the text. The 'Further References' section lists helpful books, organizations, and other resources. The 'Even Further References' section includes other supporting studies not specifically noted in the text.

More companies are developing general and specialized enzyme products as this area of health care expands. Enzymes are very specific in how they work, so getting the right enzymes for the right use is key to success. When companies and product brands are given as examples representing specific enzyme categories, I followed the format of listing either products or companies alphabetically as appropriate. The selected examples are known to be effective representations of specific categories. It is not possible to list every single product available.

I try to update information in enzyme knowledge and products with subsequent printings to keep information as current as possible. Updates are included in this book. One example is the results found with the previous Seven Month Study based on two particular enzyme products which appeared at a certain time. Since then, similar and equivalent results have been found with several other lines of quality enzyme products. Another update is the advancements in designing enzyme products for gluten and dairy digestion. The story described in my previous book following the potential success of a particular innovation in enzyme blends to replace a gluten-free, dairy-free diet and was a good example representing technology at that time. Since then, several other products have emerged with more refinements improving the range of results seen for more people. Further innovations in enzyme products have emerged as well providing even better results for various situations. Products for inflammation and viral control are now available and also proving very effective.

Although enzyme therapy has seen tremendous success over the past decade, it is important to remember this is not due to any one person, place, or product. Rather it is the collective effort of many typical, devoted families and individuals voluntarily sharing their experiences, researching on their own, and working through their particular situations. This unique collaboration in cooperation with several commercial companies focused on enzymes has produced new alternatives in health care.

The previous book titles described some of my family's adventures in enzyme therapy. This book also includes some real-life experiences. One son's name is used specifically while the other one is referred to indirectly as each son preferred. Some of the names have been changed to protect the 'guilty.' My sons as well as a few friends may not be so keen in being directly tied to some of their escapades down the road.

My work with enzyme therapy over the years has been and continues to be on a volunteer basis. The information on enzymes contained here, observations, and tests conducted were developed independently of any product manufacturer. The guidelines contained in this document were derived from extensive research literature and thousands of volunteers who contributed their experiences. This information is not medical advice or meant to replace any medical therapy you are currently undergoing or considering. Consult your health care practitioner when making changes to your health care program.

P. S. If you have any questions or concerns for me, you can contact me through my website or email. I will try to be helpful.
www.enzymestuff.com and kd@thundersnow.com
- *Karen.*

CHAPTER 1

The Lay of the Land

Ahhhhhh! The joys of home ownership! Nothing brings up a feeling quite like what comes over you when told you need to replace your entire sewer system. And there is no getting out of it. It *must* be done. Anytime the plumbing isn't what it should be, the plumber becomes the most important person on the planet.

So the yard was dug up and a lovely pristine drainage system put in. We were left with wonderful water pipes which piped the water wonderfully . . . and a yard in need of much repair. And there was no getting out of it. The disruption was so extensive, it had to be done.

Trying to get a lawn in shape is very similar to maintaining good digestive health. A lawn is a growing, dynamic entity. So is the environment in the gut. A lawn relies on an extensive root system to give it structure and bring in nutrients. We rely on a similar system exists in the intestines. A lawn has an underlying complex microbial system as does the microbe balance in the gut. In both areas, we need to be mindful of any shift in the microbe balance from one promoting health to one working against us. Nature has a way of repeating itself. This repetition can be an advantage. The principles seen in renovating and maintaining a lawn can also help in improving and maintaining digestive health.

Assessing the damage

To put this effort of our yard restoration into perspective, you need to understand the extent of the damage. One street runs in front of our house and another along the back. In the front yard, the sewer line trenching extended from the street at least 20 feet down through the entire length of the yard to the house. Another sump pump pipe was connected from the back of our house through the entire backyard and into a drainage line under the street running behind our house.

Now, our small spot of suburbia has a steep slope in the backyard. The slope is highest in the back towards the roadway sloping abruptly downwards on one side of the yard towards the house. It flattens out near our home at the bottom. At one point at the top of the slope, it was necessary to dig the trench 30-foot deep to connect the pipe to the street sewer behind our house. To manage water flow coming down the hill (towards our house), a retaining wall was built partway across the steepest part of the slope. (I told myself it also enhanced the view and added value to the area. It did end up looking quite nice.)

As a bonus, on top of having both the front and backyards plowed up, the heavy trenching equipment destroyed the side yards too (oh well, I wanted to plant some shrubs there anyway). Our slice of the neighborhood measured almost one-third of an acre. In the end, about three-fourths of the entire area needed to be repaired.

With any huge job that appears both disturbingly deep and wide, organizing it into manageable subtasks can make it easier to deal with. The first thing I did was assess the damage . . . er . . . I mean, look for opportunities to improve the landscaping. Dealing with the big ticket items first, we had sod laid over the refilled trenches in the front and back yards, and other more seriously damaged areas. This instant-lawn would prevent soil washing down the slopes and stabilize the barren areas. Sod needs to be kept moist with regular watering so it will survive and ultimately anchor into the earth below. This job of keeping the sod wet is not hard but it takes tedious persistence because sod can dry out quickly and die.

The second task was to seed the rest of the extensive amount of exposed ground. Besides the actual trenching, the nearby areas were damaged where the excess dirt had been dumped and the vehicles had trod. A third part involved replacing the bushes uprooted by the trenching in front of the house. Another job was fixing the yard on the two sides of the house. A final step was putting down mulch. Mulch, mulch, and more mulch. Mulching everything down can greatly reduce the workload long-term. And I am all for reducing the long-term workload. Mulch is my friend.

The plan was to work most of the summer and finish up by mid-fall. I don't mind yard work, and I studied agricultural science in college. So I had some idea of what was involved and the plan was sound. But you know what they say about best-laid plans.

Assessing natural similarities

Of all the plans I have had in life, working with digestive health was not one of them. I got into the area of digestive health more by accident than by choice. No, more by need. Personal health issues in my family, particularly the pervasive developmental delays of our sons, was the driving force that landed me in the situation of pouring over health literature, internet sites, and doctors' evaluations. Those who are familiar with my previous books and with my postings in the enzyme discussion group since 2001 are quite aware of how insanely difficult it can be to struggle with digestive health. And all the problems associated with it. Not just physical gut problems, but the behavior problems it brings in children and the general disruption it inflicts on one's daily life.

What I planned on was working with soils and plants, nurturing things to grow. You know, getting close to nature and all that stuff. My primary area of study was soil fertility and plant nutrition. I really enjoyed the science, especially the practical aspects of getting things to work in real life.

Agriculture is an applied science. The theories and techniques need to hold up under real-life conditions. Even if something works well in a laboratory, if actual farmers cannot apply the research to produce a decent crop under actual field conditions, it is back to the drawing board. The application of science needs to achieve a goal.

So too was my interest in digestive enzymes. I had very practical goals. I wanted to improve the health of my sons as well as myself. I wanted my migraines to end, or at least lessen. I wanted my older son to be able to function independently without so much pain. My younger son was plagued with extensive digestive problems since infancy. For him, we hoped he could simply eat food of some kind, get some bit of nutrition out of it, and not be in such digestive distress all the time. The many other families I came in contact with pursuing enzyme therapy also wanted to improve the health of their families or themselves. The focus was on getting results.

The challenge of getting digestive enzymes to actually work under real-life conditions was inherently interesting to me, especially since there was a black hole where that sort of information should have been. Guidelines for using digestive enzymes were practically non-existent. Again, it was a critical need that drove the effort to develop practical usage guidelines. And given that enzymes in general are a basic aspect of applied soil and plant science, I was both familiar and comfortable with the overall topic of enzymes.

After working with the entire issue of digestive enzymes and nutrient absorption in the gut for awhile, I kept thinking how the digestive process seemed very familiar. Very, very familiar. Not just the idea or chemistry but the actual visual picture of what was happening. Soon, it became clear.

My thesis project in graduate school centered around examining how changes in the soil environment affected root growth and nutrient uptake, and thus, plant growth overall. It included greenhouse studies as well as field studies with different plants in multiple locations over multiple years. I had the - ahem - 'interesting' job of digging up, counting, and measuring root growth in addition to tracking other measurements of soil and plant changes. (Although slavery was banished, I sometimes wondered if it didn't linger on through the use of graduate students.)

Look at this image:

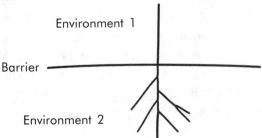

Let's say the horizontal line represents a barrier of some kind separating two different environments. We can also see that the vertical line crossing the barrier is going from one environment to the other. Lastly, one part of the vertical line has additional little lines extending out into one environment.

Now let's give this picture some functions. The vertical line can actually be a tube of some kind. And the little lines can be little tubes through which fluids or substances can move. What happens if the following labels are added to the picture?

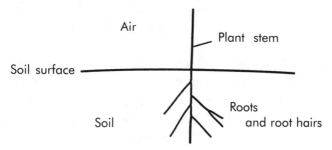

The roots and smaller root hairs extend out into the soil environment taking up available nutrients and water. These nutrients are absorbed up through the roots, into the stem, past the soil surface, and dispersed to the various parts of the plant where they are needed. The green leaves pull in carbon dioxide and manufacture carbohydrates for the plant through the process of photosynthesis. These carbohydrates are sent down through the plant and to the roots to promote root growth. These same carbohydrates end up being a critical part of animal and human survival, supplying both nutrition and energy. Without root growth, no nutrients or raw materials can be absorbed and available for plant growth.

Roots are limited to taking up nutrients that are available to them in their immediate environment. If the nutrients are three feet away, or even three inches out of reach, they will not be absorbed and used by the plant. So nutrient availability becomes a huge part of plant nutrition. Soil pH, temperature, moisture, and other factors also influence root cell reactions. and other factors. In addition, a variety of microbes live in the soil helping break down organic matter, assisting with nutrient uptake, and interacting with the roots.

Now, let's look at the previous image, keeping the structure and functions the same, but adding different labels.

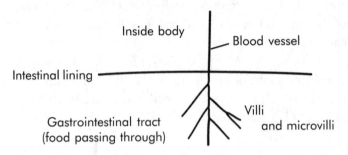

The villi and the smaller microvilli are the structures in the gut that extend into the intestinal tract and absorb any available nutrients and water passing through there. These nutrients are absorbed through the villi cells, into the bloodstream, past the intestinal barrier, and dispersed to the various parts of the body where they are needed.

Like the root cells, the villi cells are limited to taking up nutrients that are available to them in their immediate environment. And like in the soil environment, there is an active microbial community at work in the gut influencing what goes on there.

Overall plant health is in large part a product of the health of the root-soil interface. When there are nutrient deficiencies in the soil, the plant suffers. In the gut, the microvilli cells also respond to their immediate environment, the intestinal environment, which then impacts the entire body. The health of the physical body is significantly influenced by the health of the villi-intestine interface. When there are nutrient deficiencies in the intestinal environment, the body suffers.

While there are differences in plant root function and how the villi work in the intestines, there are many similarities. Looking at how a healthy root environment functions can assist in working with digestive health. Both systems strongly impact the health and growth of the organism. Both have complex communities of microbial life which can either be beneficial or harmful. Both are affected by non-nutrient factors such as fiber and biofilms. And both systems rely heavily on digestive enzymes.

Where does dirt come from?

Digestive enzymes function pretty much the same in soils and plants as they do in animals and humans - they break down organic matter. Organic matter is a compound that contains carbon as an essential element, and is derived from a living organism. The organism may be dead or in some stage of decay, but it was living at some point.

What is the difference between rock and soil? As rock breaks down through weathering processes into small mineral particles, plant and animal organic matter then mixes in with the mineral particles to form soil. This organic matter from the degraded living organisms is what differentiates rock or raw minerals from soil. The materials from the organic matter are required to sustain new life growing in the soil.

Besides plant life, soils sustain bacteria, fungi, algae, microscopic animals, and other animals like earthworms. All of these organisms living in the soil facilitate the digestion of organic matter, mixing the material up through their actions, enhancing the soil structure, and making soil minerals more available through chemical and physical reactions. Burrowing by worms and larger organisms leave channels for air and water to flow through.

Different types of soil have different amounts and types of organic matter and minerals. This leads to variations in nutrient availability, structure, moisture levels, and other functions. As organic matter decomposes, it can turn into a substance called humus. Humus acts sort of like a glue that binds smaller soil particles together. Peat is another type of soil heavy in organic matter. Sandy soils have relatively little organic matter. Each type of soil can support life, but it needs to be managed differently based on its own unique behaviors, properties, and 'personality.' Understanding the nuances of the environment you are working with helps you to be able to manipulate it so you get the results you want.

Similarly, individuals can have vastly different biology influencing their intestinal environments. The solution for optimal gut health will require each individual to find the variations suitable for their situation based on general themes. Even the members of my small family all benefited from a slightly different enzyme and health program, even though we all followed the same basic principles.

Determining the problem

Gads, those days were so hard! When our older son was contorting in pain. When he was screaming uncontrollably and none of the specialists knew what to do. When he would withdraw sharply into himself and not interact with others. When he would bang his head on the floor over and over for hours on end. When I would fight through my own migraine pain to try to find a solution for his torment. I couldn't afford the luxury of nursing my own head pain. Not that anything had ever been able to relieve it anyway. Gads, those days were so hard.

I shake those memories away as I look out on the destruction we once called a yard. This restoration project was a bit overwhelming actually. I remembered how overwhelming the whole situation with my sons had been then too. I had lived with my own constant migraines for so long I was used to the pain that existed with every breath. No, it was our older son that was suffering the most at the moment. They were times of complete exasperation when everyone agreed there was a serious problem, but no one knew what to do about it. Even after he eventually was diagnosed with pervasive developmental and neurological problems, the road was not clear. The sea of conflicting options made *me* want to pound my head on the floor for hours.

It should have been easier with my younger son. Since his issues were more physical instead of behavioral, it should have been easier for some pediatric specialist to diagnose whatever was causing his chronic gagging reflux, his refusal to eat, and his chronic bowel problems. But after years of dealing with his gut problems, what should have been just wasn't going to be.

Eventually, solutions came. Bit by bit. Following a process of analysis, research, application, then revise and refine, and try again, it was possible to hone in on each of our problems and deal with it.

Determining the cause of a health problem can be difficult and tedious. A bit of detective work is usually needed. Generally there are visible symptoms letting you know there is a problem. Symptoms can be behavioral, cognitive, or physical. However, the difficulty with biology is that multiple problems can often cause similar symptoms.

Let's say you are growing corn and one day you see the corn leaves are turning yellow instead of staying a deep healthy green. The color of the leaves going from green to yellow is a symptom. One symptom. It can provide guidance about what the problem is, but it does not tell you exactly what is wrong. 'Turning yellow' is just one sign that needs to be evaluated with other factors in order to determine what is really causing the plant's poor health; and consequently what actions to take. Plants 'turning yellow' could be caused by:

- Water-logged soil
- Lack of water
- Lack of nitrogen (nutrient deficiency)
- Pathogens - insects, bacteria, fungi, parasites
- Chemical injury
- Soil compaction
- Physical injury from machinery

These various causes of poor plant health require very different solutions. Notice that water-logged soil and lack of water are essentially opposite conditions involving the amount of water present, but both extremes cause plants to turn yellow. How can this be? Plant roots need both water and oxygen in balance. When water floods the soil, the spaces are filled leaving no room in the soil for oxygen. The roots are basically suffocating. When no water is present, there is plenty of oxygen but no moisture for the plant. The plants die of thirst. Either extreme causes the plant to suffer and turn yellow.

The same thing happens when evaluating intestinal health. Constipation is a symptom. A symptom potentially caused by a number of possibilities. It takes more investigation to find out what is causing the constipation, and thus, determine what you need to do to alleviate the problem.

So what to do? How does one diagnose what is going on? You can analyze the overall environment. With corn plants, you can walk the fields, assess nutrient levels, study the water drainage, examine other plants growing near the plant in question, and hunt for pathogens both above ground as well as in the soil itself. With intestinal health, you can do similar evaluations. You can write down any symptoms, including physical, behavioral, and cognitive changes. You can analyze the diet nutrient levels, check for environment irritants, note physical activity, look at sleep patterns, and other possibilities. Keeping a daily diary of foods, behaviors, and symptoms may help reveal patterns that would not otherwise be detected.

Next, look at the micro-environment to the degree you are able or comfortable with. With plants, you can run a soil analysis to determine the nutritional profile of the soil as well as physical factors affecting nutrient availability. You can also analyze some of the plant leaves to determine nutritional levels. Similar types of tests are available for human health. Nutritional analysis can tell you if there are certain nutrient deficiencies. There are tests for determining bacteria, yeast overgrowth, and viruses. Unfortunately, though, many of these tests are not 100% accurate. Tests on living things can only take a snapshot of a certain state of health at a certain period in time. They cannot in and of themselves tell you what is causing the problem or what to do about it. But tests can sometimes provide another piece of information.

A reasonable guide to determine what tests to run is ask what the results will tell you and what you will do once you get the results back. Also, the accuracy of the test needs to be fairly high. Sometimes many expensive tests are run only to receive multiple papers and unexplained numbers back. The results are not translated into a course of action, and you are no closer to a solution than you were before all the tests were run. It is worth spending a little time investigating any test you are considering to get a clear understanding of how you can translate any results into a course of action before doing the tests.

There are no tests for determining absolutely if you would benefit from digestive enzymes or not. Fortunately, it is relatively inexpensive and quick to just try enzymes and see if they help. A few tests that look at various aspects of digestion in general are available, which you can consider with your health practitioner's guidance.

Eventually, you should be able to narrow down the problem to a few possibilities. Then you need to try something appropriate for one of the possibilities and monitor the results. Then take what you learned from those results - both good and bad - revise the plan, and try again. Then monitor those results, revise, and go again. This is a standard part of working with individual biology. Even if you are working closely with a health practitioner, this is the same process they generally use whether or not it is obvious.

Keep in mind that as much can often be learned by something not working as when something is successful. Just because a measure did not bring the hoped for results does not mean it was a total failure. Or completely without value. Unsuccessful measures can help you rule possibilities out. Or point out what might be the next best step.

When I was trying to figure out if my son had an intestinal pathogen, I first tried a yeast treatment. No response. I tried something for parasites. No response. When I then tried an antibiotic for bacteria, there was a big response. Bingo! Now I knew to focus on bacteria and problems associated with that type of pathogen.

With digestive enzymes, you may experience many benefits but still have a few remaining symptoms or food intolerances left. These 'leftovers' can be helpful in pointing out possible next steps. For example, you may find that many foods can be added back in with enzymes except for certain ones. Looking at common factors in this group of leftover foods may lead you to find that artificial colorings or amines are a problem. Or you may experience a very dramatic reaction to fiber digesting enzymes and see certain stool characteristics indicating a possible *Candida* problem. In this way, starting enzymes early can provide guidance to your overall health care program.

And so it begins . . .

This steady process of trying something, monitoring results, revising and moving on is one of persistence . . . tedious persistence. Just like watering sod to keep it alive. The process may produce quicker results for some than others, but not seeing quick results does not mean you 'did something wrong.' You may simply have a different unique situation that requires more time and effort.

I watered all the sod in our yard several times a day. The sod on top of the back slope grew into the rich black soil there within a few weeks. The sod in the front yard containing less nutrient-rich soil and more sand blended into the ground within a few months. However, the sod put down at the base of slope in the back was constantly flooded even though I applied less water there than the other two spots. The standing water was drowning the sod, slowly killing it off. After some time, I pulled up part of the sod and examined the underlying soil. It was a clay pan, hard as a rock. The water was literally standing on top of that barrier. The barrier also made it nearly impossible for the little roots to burrow into it. Drat. This was not part of the plan. Need to adjust and adapt. Sod is not going to work here. I moved the sod from that area to another spot where the soil had better drainage while considering what to do with that clay pan.

Understanding the soil types involved helped explain why there were such different responses even though the sod applied was exactly the same. Similarly, knowing how the gut is structured and the variations within it may help you understand the reactions and results you see with the measures you try.

CHAPTER 2

Location, Location, Location
– The Gut-brain Connection

The range of health improvements using digestive enzyme therapy has been both deep and wide. My sons both benefited immensely even though they had different 'issues.' Now, I could see how a digestive aid could help a digestive problem. That is pretty straightforward. It was pretty easy to understand how enzymes greatly helped the son with the substantial digestive problems. However, it was not so easy to see why digestive enzymes would help my other son with all the intense behavior problems. This son was struggling to deal with daily life. Interestingly, he showed no digestive problems at all! We had no reason to even consider digestive aids. Yet he improved significantly with enzymes. Why would this happen? Why would digestive enzymes help end chronic head-banging? Improve sleep? Why would enzymes help improve his grades and getting along with other kids at school?

The same thing happens with adults too. It is understandable how enzymes help relieve reflux, food intolerances, or constipation. But why do enzymes help adults increase their productivity at work, end fatigue, and improve mood, clear thinking, and auto-immune problems?

The answer appears to lie in how the gut is laid out physically. The geography of the small intestine in particular holds the clues. It is a matter of location, location, location.

The digestive system functions beginning with the first thought of food. Food goes in the mouth, down the throat, into the stomach, through the small intestines, through the large intestine (colon), and anything left is eliminated out through the anus. There are a lot of opportunities for food breakdown during this process through both mechanical and chemical methods. The complete process is detailed in Chapter 3 of *Enzymes for Autism/Digestive Health*.

Digestive System

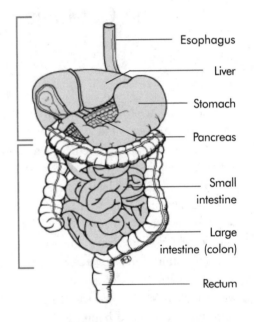

• Nutrients not absorbed in stomach and upper GI tract
• Lower pH
• Pancreatic enzymes are destroyed in this area
• Plant and microbial enzymes actively provide extra pre-digestion of food before reaching the small intestine

• Nutrients absorbed in intestines and lower GI tract
• Higher pH
• All enzymes active in this region

Esophagus

Liver

Stomach

Pancreas

Small intestine

Large intestine (colon)

Rectum

Digestion includes the total process from when food first goes into your mouth until it is either absorbed into the body or is expelled out the other end as waste. Digestion can become impaired at any point in the digestive process. You may experience different symptoms depending on where in the gastrointestinal tract there is a problem. It may be helpful to map out where in the digestive process you are experiencing problems. Once these are marked off, look at how the injured part affects the rest of the digestive process past this point.

For example, you may have low stomach acid for an assortment of reasons. Since stomach acid is needed to trigger the release of bicarbonate and digestive enzymes from the pancreas, having low stomach acid will reduce the amount of digestive enzymes released from the pancreas. This can lead to less overall enzyme activity in the small intestine, which can lead to more undigested food reaching the colon, which can lead to colon problems or bacteria overgrowth. If, on the other hand, you have a colon issue, only the colon and rectum areas may be affected. The rest of the digestive process taking place before the colon may be fine.

The great gains in enzyme therapy in the past decades are due in part to new innovations in developing enzyme products. Food is not absorbed in the stomach. The stomach is an area of initial digestion before being absorbed in the intestines. Pancreatic enzyme supplements are like the enzymes our own pancreas produces. Pancreatic enzymes are not active in the digestive tract until the food reaches the small intestine where the pH is higher.

Plant and microbial-derived enzymes, however, are active throughout the entire digestive tract. These enzymes have greater stability in the stomach environment. This means plant and microbial-derived enzymes have significantly more time to digest food in the stomach. They can work a good 60 to 90 minutes or more, *before* the food reaches the small intestine where it can be absorbed. This 'pre-digestion' with these types of enzymes minimizes adverse reactions further along in the digestive tract. In a leaky gut situation, thoroughly digested food reaching the intestines is less likely to provoke an adverse reaction even if it crosses an injured gut lining inappropriately. The food is not in the larger forms which provoke adverse reactions.

Structure of the small intestine

Once the food reaches the small intestine, enzymes from both the pancreas and the intestinal lining are active (any supplemental enzymes would be active here as well). Three major systems are interconnected throughout the intestines. It is this physical layout that can explain much of the success with digestive enzymes, both with digestive problems and behavior issues in children and adults.

Location of the absorptive surfaces

Once the contents of the stomach pass into the small intestine, absorption is possible. Food, supplements, and medications are only meant to be absorbed if they are in the proper form. Otherwise, the contents should be screened out.

To get a good idea of what the small intestine looks like and how it functions, think of a bath towel laid out flat with all those absorbent loops pointing up. Now, if you roll that towel up into a tube with all the loops inside, this is a good model of the small intestine. If you send fluids down through the tube, those absorbent loops would be soaking up what they could as the fluid passed through. Any larger substances would not be taken up through the loops.

The villi structures in the small intestine are like the loops of the towel. They absorb nutrients from the small intestine as the stomach contents pass through. Each of the numerous villi are covered with more finer loops known as microvilli. All the folding and looping vastly increases the surface area in the gut for maximum absorption of nutrients.

Cross-section of the Small Intestine

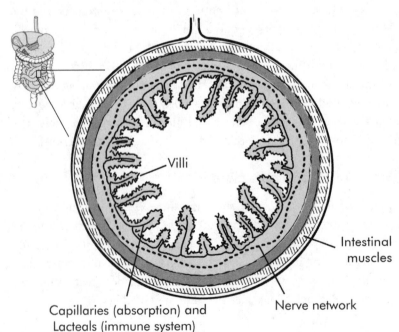

Villi

Intestinal muscles

Capillaries (absorption) and Lacteals (immune system)

Nerve network

Another way to think of villi is like plant roots extending into the soil absorbing water and nutrients. Roots do not absorb everything they come into contact with, only certain substances in the appropriate form. Root hairs are similar to microvilli. They increase the absorptive surface area entending into the nutritional environment.

If you have a very lush towel with lots of long, dense, plush loops, this towel would be very absorbent. It would properly absorb moisture while screening out substances that are too large or not in the proper form. This is similar to a healthy intestinal tract and good nutrient absorption. Now, think of a low quality towel. The type you may have if you bought it for, say, one dollar. You know, the type that has about three loops per square inch? It does not absorb very well because there are fewer, more scraggly loops.

Villi in the Small Intestine

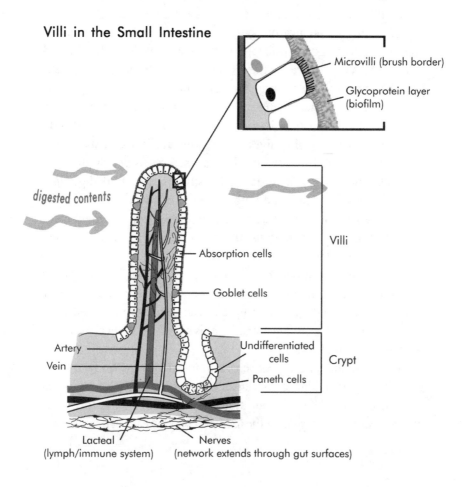

If the towel gets worn out, torn, or damaged, the threads become looser and the towel may even have holes. This towel cannot properly soak up moisture or screen out the wrong substances. A damaged towel is similar to a damaged intestinal tract or leaky gut situation. Intestinal damage leads to poor absorption (malabsorption), nutrient deficiencies, and food intolerances among other problems.

The same happens with plant roots. A healthy extensive root system supports good plant growth. A damaged root system compromises the plant's health. Too much root damage leads to plant death.

Location of the immune system

The majority of the immune system lies in the gut running along the entire gastrointestinal tract. If a substance crosses into the body when it should be screened out, the immune system is located right there in the gut lining to pounce on these intruders. There are a variety of immune system agents available. Lacteals are inside each villi and secretory IgA is produced in the crypt regions of the villi. Paneth cells produce an assortment of antimicrobial compounds.

Even if you eat healthy nutritional food, if there is damaged tissue or 'leaks' in the intestinal barrier, particles can cross into the body before they are thoroughly digested. Unfortunately, the immune system is not clever enough to identify these substances as poorly digested food and send them back inside the digestive tract for more digesting. It only knows the compound is not meant to be there and sounds the alarm. The immune system acts and may even inappropriately mark these compounds as hazardous substances. This is a prime way food intolerances develop.

As the immune system becomes busier and busier attacking food compounds, its resources are diverted from the true harmful invaders. The immune system can ramp up and run at a more elevated level attacking everything. But maintaining this hyper-active level over time stresses the entire body.

Once the immune system senses an invader in the body, it locks onto the compound like a policeman handcuffing a crook forming an immune complex. The immune system police then try to process the 'bad guy' out of the system. If the immune complex cannot be processed out quickly enough, they can build up in the body and lead to a variety of autoimmune conditions.

Location of the nervous system

Along with the location of the absorptive surfaces and the location of the immune system, a major network of nerves runs thoughout the gastrointestinal structure. The enteric nervous system (ENT) is similar to the central nervous system (CNS) and communicates with it. Whenever there is damage in the gut, nerves are tripped signaling various reactions. The nerve cells can also be directly damaged along with other types of cells in the gut.

Existing along with these nerves are neurotransmitters. Researchers estimate a good 90% of all serotonin receptors are located in the gut (Gershon 1998). Serotonin is one of several neurotransmitters that influence mood. Serotonin promotes calmness and overall well-being. Someone with an injured gut would likely have problems with serotonin due to the location of serotonin in the gut. You would expect someone with serotonin problems to suffer depression, moodiness, agitation, anxiety, and perhaps even hyperness or aggression.

Serotonin is also a precursor to melatonin, which is important for good restful sleep. You would expect a person having problems with serotonin levels to also have problems with sleep. This is how gut problems can cause problems with mood, sleep, and neurological function. Gut health is interrelated with sensory processing function. A person who is sleep-deprived is hyper-sensitive to lights, sounds, smells, textures, and other sensory inputs. The quality of sleep influences the perception of pain and how we react to sensory inputs. Thus, it is logical that a person with gastrointestinal problems or sleep problems would have also have sensory processing problems.

It is interesting to note that one of the most successful classes of medications for depression, neurological problems, sleep disorders, and an assortment of children's behavior problems (including autism conditions) is the class of SSRIs, the selective serotonin reuptake inhibitors. I found out when my younger son was diagnosed with irritable bowel symdrome (IBS) that the SSRIs tend to be successful with IBS and other colon problems.

So now we see a direct relationship between intestinal damage and nerve reactions. A digestive problem can lead directly to a neurological problem due to the structural relationships in the gut. A nerve problem can manifest in all sorts of ways. Examples include migraines, odd behaviors, sleep disorders, and muscle spasms. The nerves in the gut can also influence the muscle fluxes in the gut, such as peristalsis which moves food contents through the intestines (or not!). A point of injury in the gut also directly provokes the immune system into action and interferes with nutrient absorption all because of the geographical location of all these structures.

Enzymes of the intestinal lining

Focusing closer on the villi structures, a single layer of cells covers the outer surface. These surface cells are mainly absorptive cells with microvilli extending out of the cell membranes into the intestinal cavity. The microvilli cells produce some important enzymes and assist with food breakdown. The enzyme proteins are anchored in the villi-microvilli cell membranes. As food compounds come into contact with the anchored enzymes, the enzymes act to break the compounds apart. The end products are then taken into the absorptive cells by various absorption mechanisms.

Goblet cells are also interspersed on the outer surface layer. Goblet cells secrete mucus. Mucus serves several functions including trapping and carrying off various substances, protecting the gut cells and overall body. The mucus helps protect the gut tissue against physical stress and chemical damage.

The primary intestinal enzymes are disaccharidases and certain peptidases. Disaccharidases break down complex carbohydrates. These are the sugars and 'carbs' found in starchy foods. These are also the carbohydrates that yeast or bacteria can use for growth should the food not be absorbed. The main disaccharidases in the intestinal lining are sucrase, lactase, maltase, and isomaltase. Lactase is an enzyme that digests lactose, or milk sugar. A person who is lactose intolerant does not have enough of the enzyme lactase for proper digestion. Lack of lactase may be due to genetics or because of damage to the cells that produce lactase. Simple sugars are called monosaccharides and can be absorbed directly without requiring intestinal enzymes for further breakdown. The three most common simple sugars are glucose (also known as blood sugar), galactose (found in dairy), and fructose (found in honey and fruits).

Peptidases are enzymes that break down peptides. A peptide is any fragment or chunk derived from a protein. There are multitudes of peptide types in all sizes, shapes, and chemical makeup. There are multitudes of corresponding peptidases to break the peptides down further as well. One of these villi cell peptidases is a very important one known as DPP-IV (dipeptyl dipeptidase IV). DPP-IV describes an enzyme activity which breaks down a particularly stubborn bond found in casein (a protein in dairy), gluten (a protein in small cereal grains), and possibly other protein containing foods.

If the villi cells are damaged or missing, these intestinal enzymes will not be available to break down foods. Hold your hand out open in front of you. Your fingers represent the villi. If you start to curl your hand very slowly into a fist, imagine how this illustrates progressive gut injury. With more and more damage, more enzyme activity is lost. We would expect someone losing these enzymes to have difficulty digesting dairy, grains, and complex carbohydrates . . . the food types relying on these intestinal enzymes the most for thorough breakdown.

The casein-free, gluten-free diet (GFCF diet) is based on eliminating any foods requiring DPP IV activity. Most people, particularly children, eat diets high in these foods and so these may be noticed first as problem foods. The popularity of low-carb and specific carbohydrate diets in the last decade may be related to the loss of the disaccharidases caused by gut injury - and a hint that intestinal health in the general population is less than optimal.

The good news is that it works both ways. Take your fist and now slowly unravel it. As the gut heals, the villi tissue cells can grow back and the ability to produce lactase, disaccharidases, and peptidases can return. How the villi cells grow is very interesting.

Villi cells are formed from undifferentiated stem cells located near the base of the villi in the crypt region. From these undifferentiated cells, goblet and absorptive cells form, divide off, and march up the side of the villi in single file to the tip of the villi. At the tip, they are eventually sloughed off in the digestive tract and eliminated in waste.

Physiology textbooks give the time for cells to grow from the basal undifferentiated cells to the tip of the villi as five days. It takes about five days for the cells to start developing at the base of the villi, make their way up side of the villi, and reach the tip of the villi before sloughing off. This correlates nicely with the trend of an upset stomach running a course of four or five days; or the recommendation to allow four to five days for adverse reactions to subside when you remove dairy when it is thought to be a problem food. Also note that a rotation diet is structured so different foods are eaten over a four to five day period. Hmmmm . . . a pattern emerges.

Physiology textbooks say it takes three to four weeks, or 21 to 30 days, for complete turnover of all the gastrointestinal tissue cells. That is, it takes nearly one month for damaged dead cells to be replaced with newer cells throughout the digestive tract. This correlates with the timeframe commonly seen for adjustments to resolve when you start enzymes. It is also the time frame commonly given to allow for detoxification cleanses to run their course. Extensions of allowing up to six weeks are also common in more serious cases.

Tales from the crypt

Paneth cells form in the bottom of the villi structure in the crypt region. The exact nature and function of Paneth cells is not completely understood; however, it is known these cells produce several compounds that are protective in nature. Paneth cells produce the enzyme lysozyme that works against harmful microbes. This is an immediate mechanism to help prevent dysbiosis and disease in the digestive tract.

Within the Paneth cells are specialized proteins known as metallothioneins (MT). MT proteins act like heavy metal magnets that bind up heavy metals. MT proteins are found in many tissues throughout the plant and animal kingdoms.

In the gut, these proteins are responsible for sequestering or removing harmful metals so the heavy metals cannot enter the body where they could cause all types of havoc. If MT-containing cells are physically located in the gut lining, then it is understandable that when the intestinal tissue becomes injured, for any reason, these MT proteins would also be damaged, not present, or otherwise unable to function properly. Gut injury can thus lead to poor heavy metal detoxification, metal toxicity, or damage in the body due to metal accumulation. It is also reasonable that healing an injured digestive tract would restore the MT-producing cells and return proper detoxification function in the gut environment. (Danielson, Ohi, and Huang 1982; Mullins and Fuentealba 1998)

Other functions of MT in the gut include regulating stomach acid pH, and taste and texture discrimination by the tongue. Low levels of MT may lead to problems in these other areas as well. (Masters *et al* 1994; Qauife *et al* 1994)

MT proteins also have an important role in regulating trace metal metabolism, including the critical function of maintaining a healthy balance between copper and zinc. Excess accumulation of either element can lead to toxicity problems. Copper toxicity is associated with many types of neurological problems. The Pfeiffer Treatment Center (PTC) has worked on the MT, zinc, and detoxification issue for several years. This organization found that most people with autism, ADHD, and related conditions have excessively high copper levels and very low zinc. Pfeiffer's program focuses on bringing the high copper and low zinc back into balance with a fair amount of success.

The Paneth cells in the villi crypts are also reservoirs of zinc. The high zinc concentrations may be due to this element's association with the MT proteins. Each MT molecule in the gut requires seven atoms of zinc to function. When zinc is deficient, MT cannot function and, thus, heavy metals that should be bound up instead travel freely in the body where they can potentially cause harm. In an interesting loop, the presence of heavy metals, mainly the heavy metal zinc, can influence how much MT is synthesized, assembled, and activated.

Low levels of zinc limit how much MT is created in the body. And this lack of MT will allow excess heavy metals to accumulate. Copper is a heavy metal that competes with zinc. If copper accumulates, it can drive a zinc deficiency even further. A vicious cycle develops with less zinc available to trigger MT production leading to more copper accumulation which then continues to lower zinc concentrations.

As zinc is added, the excess copper level declines and MT starts to form. As the MT forms, heavy metals begin to be removed properly. This is a process which should be monitored by an appropriate health care practitioner. You should not dash out and start wolfing down mega-doses of zinc. Too much zinc too quickly can cause some adverse reactions if copper is mobilized too quickly into the system.

Zinc, then, becomes critically important in the formation and proper function of MT and thus, heavy metal removal in the intestinal lining.

In a reasonably healthy system, a certain amount of stress can also increase the amount of MT produced. This is apparently one of the body's protective measures. 'Stress' can be anything from physical injury to a microbial infection to emotional anxiety. However, the negatives of too much stress, particularly over prolonged periods of time, can outweigh any short-term gains from moderate amounts of stress. And there may be no gains if overall health is compromised to begin with. (Andrews 2000; Cousins 1985; Davis and Cousins 2000; Riordan and Vallee 1991)

Zinc - Key healer in the gut

Besides its role in MT function, research shows the integrity of the gut suffers when zinc is deficient, including observed increases in inflammation and ulcers. Fortunately, supplementing zinc enhances cell production in the gut and facilitates the reversal of intestinal damage. (Duff and Ettarh 2002)

The animal with a digestive tract most similar to humans is the pig. Piglets commonly suffer a decline in health during weaning and are very susceptible to disease during this time. Often diarrhea or bacterial infections such as *Clostridia* set in. Interestingly, these are conditions also seen in human infants and toddlers. In plants, roots may go through a type of 'shock' when seedlings are transplanted from a nursery environment to another spot.

An abrupt change in the nutritional environment can lead to abrupt changes in the structures responsible for pulling nutrition into a plant or animal. Changes may be beneficial, or not. If you are aware these changes may occur, you can take steps to manage them to minimize the negatives and maximize the benefits.

When transplanting, plants are often 'conditioned' by slowly changing their growing environment to prepare them for the transition to the new area. This practice greatly increases the survival and subsequent growth rate of the seedlings.

With children, one management practice is the standard recommendation to add in foods new to a young child's diet slowly and one at a time. If you are switching from one diet to another diet abruptly, you may experience an uncomfortable adjustment period in the very beginning as the gut environment shifts in response to the nutritional change. Changing gradually over the course of a couple weeks may minimize discomfort or problems.

A common practice in the swine industry is to add higher levels of zinc to piglet nursery diets to promote growth during the weaning transition. Studies indicate added zinc may help by producing deeper crypts and greater total thickness in the small intestine. These changes increase the total area available for nutrient absorption and improve gut health. Giving zinc also increases the concentrations of intestinal metallothionein (MT proteins). (Carlson *et al* 1998; Hill *et al* 2000; Szczurek, Bjornsson, and Taylor 2001)

A study by Tran *et al* (2003) looked specifically at zinc, metallothionein levels, and gut integrity. The study examined the effects of zinc, bovine whey-derived growth factor extract (WGFE), and zinc plus WGFE on induced gut damage in rats. The researchers assessed gut histology and intestinal permeability after testing for 10 days.

The results showed the addition of WGFE reduced intestinal damage and a therapeutic dose of zinc enhanced recovery. The treatment also improved intestinal permeability (leaky gut). In combination, zinc and WGFE hastened repair of gut damage. Measurements taken on days five and seven showed gut metallothionein concentrations throughout the intestines were significantly higher in rats fed supplemental zinc than those not receiving zinc.

Another study demonstrated how supplemental zinc significantly enhanced MT production throughout the body when piglets were given zinc for several weeks around the weaning period (Carlson, Hill, and Link 1999) .

These results confirm the relationship between supplementing zinc and increasing MT levels in the gut. They also verify zinc supplements can assist with healing intestinal damage within days of starting the zinc. Supplementing with zinc, and including zinc-rich foods in the diet, are good fundamental yet inexpensive ways to repair intestinal damage and assist with reducing the body's excess heavy metal burden.

An interesting observation is that adding zinc supplements can often resolve a problem known as the 'chewies.' The chewies refers to a problem in some children, particular those with sensory problems or developmental delays, where the child is constantly chewing on non-food items - shirt collars or sleeves, furniture, toys, wallpaper, sand, or whatever. The child may have oral fixations or may be hypersensitive to textures and tastes in foods. The child may be ultra-picky to certain foods, perhaps even gagging on certain foods for no apparent reason.

Recall that a function of MT in the gastrointestinal tract is to regulate taste and texture discrimination. If MT is deficient, this ability to properly discern food textures and non-foods may not be functioning appropriately. Zinc supplementation is a common fix for the 'chewies' problem. *Note:* if adding zinc does not resolve the chewing problem, try magnesium, and then other minerals such as calcium or a mineral blend. Related information is on page 26.

Other research found zinc supplemented to weaned pigs helped maintain the stability of the the intestinal microflora during the first two weeks after weaning when stress is at its maximum (Katouli *et al* 1999; Case and Carlson 2002). The practical application for humans is that adding zinc to a probiotic program may improve the colonization of the probiotics. Zinc may help either by facilitating the activity of the probiotics or by removing harmful pathogens.

Understanding the structure of the gut, particularly the relationship between features in the small intestine can go a long way in explaining the how digestive enzymes, and digestive health in general, produce the great variety of improvements seen with enzymes. These relationships help explain why people taking enzymes see so many improvements in behavior, physical symptoms, neurological problems, and autoimmune conditions besides the more clear-cut benefits in digestive and bowel problems.

CHAPTER 3

Where Do Enzymes Fit In?

My brother's keeper

Matthew and his brother were trudging through the lawn care section of the lumber shop. They were supposed to be waiting at the mulch section while I brought the van around to load it. We needed *a lot* of mulch.

"Hey, look at this!" said Matthew grabbing his brother's arm and pulling him over to a side aisle. He had spotted some outdoor fixtures.

"Look at *what?*" his brother asked, annoyed at being suddenly jerked.

"We can use this! We *need* this. Let's ask Mom if we can buy it!" The object of Matthew's newfound desire was a black iron shepherd's crook used to hang a bird feeder or plant basket on in the yard.

"What do you want *that* for?" his brother asked impatiently. He knew they were supposed to be at the mulch and didn't want to get into trouble . . . again. Matthew's 'distractions' and 'ideas' tended to produce interesting results.

"A *weapon!*" Matthew was just beaming!

This did not sound good. Their mother frowned on that sort of thing. But the idea of a weapon had a certain allure to it.

"How is that a weapon?" Matthew's brother asked. He was not sure how this was supposed to work.

"Well, when the bad guys come to attack us, I can jump out of my bedroom window, roll across the deck with a ninja scream, grab this out of the ground, and whack their legs out from under them. Then, we can pin them to the ground with this hook part," exclaimed Matthew, getting louder and more animated as he explained his obviously brilliant plan. He was acting out each motion of the story in exaggerated detail until he ended triumphantly by demonstrating how the gardening hook would fit nicely around someone's neck by stretching it over his brother's head.

"Cut it out!" his brother yelped, jerking out of the trap and bumping into a display of gardening tools. Gads, how irritating! He greatly disliked being suddenly strangled by the shepherd's crook in the middle of the store. Not that he wanted to be assaulted by a lawn ornament anywhere, mind you.

He moaned in frustration at Matthew, "Can't you act somewhat regular at least half the time?!"

"Awwwhh," Matthew asked sporting the best puppy-dog face he could muster, "What fun would that be?" He didn't mean to make his brother mad. He just got excited as the ideas flooded into his head.

"You're crazy!" his brother whined.

"And that's what you love about me, right?" Matthew whipped out brightly as he straightened up the disrupted display.

Matthew's brown-haired brother rolled his eyes, a small smile emerging. The tension left as funny thoughts of their past adventures pranced around in his head. His brother was right, although he would never willingly admit it. Matthew could be frustrating at times, but he did keep things lively. Never a dull moment with him around. It's just Matthew's rapid fire brain could wear you out at times. As could the rapid fire chatter that went with it. He pulled Matthew's arm.

"C'mon. We need to go." He tried to think where the mulch was. He tried to think in which direction they had been going. All this thinking was making his head hurt.

"You think too much." said Matthew as he pointed the way to the mulch.

"That's just what I was thinking."

"Thought so."

Relationships can be thought of as having a certain structure and flow with each person 'fitting in' somehow. However, the exact nature of the relationship may not be immediately apparent. The relationship between digestive enzymes and nutrition is both simple and complex.

Enzyme relationships

All enzymes are proteins that do work in nature. Enzymes are organized into general categories based on their source and function.

1. Food enzymes - occur naturally in raw food; this is what makes food rot away. If food and other organic matter did not rot or decompose in some way, we would be up to the clouds in fallen leaves and dinosaurs.

Commercial enzymes are harvested from a few particular fruits and used in health care as well as digestive aids. I refer to these as the 'fruity-enzymes.' The first two enzymes on this list are commonly used and well-researched. The latter two are used less frequently.

- Papain - from papaya
- Bromelain -from pineapple
- Actinidin - from kiwi
- Ficin - from fig

Note: If you have an allergy to one of the fruits listed, avoid taking any of these particular types of enzymes. In addition, papain is cross-listed as reactive with latex allergy because it comes from the 'latex' part of the papaya fruit.

2. Digestive enzymes - produced by living organisms. They can come from animals, humans, fish, birds, bacteria, yeast, or other such organisms. Digestive enzymes specifically break down various substances for the organism to use for nourishment. This category includes enzymes produced in the pancreas, saliva, stomach, and intestinal cells. When digestive enzyme action breaks down organic matter in our bodies, we call it 'eating food.' At times when it happens outside our bodies, such as in a compost pile, we refer to this action as rotting, decomposing, or decaying.

Enzymes sold as supplements are refined and purified from one of these digestive enzyme sources. Pancreatic enzymes, or pancreatin, come from animals, usually cattle (ox or ox bile) or swine (porcine). A variety of bacteria and fungal sources produce the enzymes commonly found in most enzyme supplements. These microbial-derived enzymes are also extensively refined and purified through a tedious process until only the enzymes remain.

Microbial-derived enzymes are often grouped together with fruit-derived enzymes and collectively referred to as 'plant enzymes' or 'vegetarian enzymes.' Pancreatic enzymes are also referred to as animal-derived enzymes or pancreatin.

3. Metabolic enzymes - produced in organisms at the cellular level on an as-needed basis. Metabolic enzymes cannot be taken as supplements. They need to be produced by the body, or the organism, internally. These enzymes are the workers in nature. They build various tissues, transfer compounds from one molecule to another, oxidize substances, reduce things, etc. There may be millions of different types of metabolic enzymes because each particular enzyme has a different job. Most of the genetic related health problems involving enzyme functions are referring to metabolic enzymes.

These three categories indicate the *source* of the enzymes. Within the second category, the category of digestive enzymes, there are two subcategories based on how the digestive enzymes are *used*. These two uses follow labeled as 2a and 2b.

> 2a. Used for food breakdown - digestive enzymes used in this way are taken with food to break foods into smaller pieces.

> 2b. Used to remove things from the body - digestive enzymes used in this way are taken between meals. Taking digestive enzymes between meals avoids enzymes being slowed down working on food. The enzymes get into the body quickly to help reduce inflammation, break down yeast or bacteria, assist with viral control elements, remove harmful plaque and fibrin, clean out immune complexes, and remove other types of assorted gunk.

What is a 'systemic' enzyme?

Pay particular attention to the term 'systemic enzymes.' The term systemic enzymes is used by individuals as well as in written material to describe both category 3, metabolic enzymes, and subcategory 2b, digestive enzymes used between meals. This makes things confusing. When talking about category 3, we are discussing enzymes working in the body at the cellular or even subcellular level (meaning metabolic enzymes or enzymes besides digestive ones). When talking about subcategory 2b, we are referring to digestive enzymes used to do cleaning and healing in the body (working in ways besides digesting food). It can be tricky to determine which category a source is referring to when using the term systemic enzymes, unless there is other supporting information to clarify the meaning.

To add to the confusion, there are some diets referred to as 'metabolic diets' which include using digestive enzymes. When you take enzyme supplements, you are not swallowing metabolic enzymes directly to improve metabolic function. However, taking digestive enzymes may improve metabolic function indirectly because:

- Improving food digestion makes nutrients more available in the body so it has the raw materials it needs to run better. The thorough digestion of protein foods can help supply the basic amino acids needed to produce metabolic enzymes. Some enzymes require co-factors, usually a mineral such as magnesium or zinc. If the mineral is not present or is deficient, the metabolic enzyme cannot function. Digestive enzymes help release these minerals from food sources.

- Improving digestion releases more energy to your body. Having more energy in the body improves cellular metabolism, lessens fatigue, and helps you function better.

- Taking enzyme supplements helps keep gunk and debris cleaned out, and pathogen levels down.

- Taking enzyme supplements to help digest your food and keep the body cleaned out means that your own metabolism does not have to spend resources doing this. Your immune system and metabolism can focus better on other areas of running the body when they are not bogged down with food digestion. This is similar to when you get really sick. The body needs all the energy and raw materials it can muster to fight off the pathogen, so you temporarily lose your appetite and lay low resting.

Digestive enzymes may be a significant help even if the fundamental problem involves a metabolic enzyme. While digestive enzymes cannot replace metabolic enzymes, they can support the body in other ways.

Sometimes a person will have a test run for levels of liver enzymes. They may get a test result back saying they have elevated liver enzymes and want to know if this means they have too many enzymes already and should not take digestive enzyme supplements. Liver enzyme levels refer to certain metabolic enzymes that work in the liver. These tests measure certain aspects of liver function. In general, 'elevated liver enzymes' indicates the liver is stressed for some reason. Digestive enzyme supplements are not related to nor do they affect liver enzymes, except possibly in a beneficial indirect way. Supplementing digestive enzymes may improve health in a way so the liver is less stressed.

Enzymes, vitamins, minerals, and other nutrients

Enzymes are not nutrients in and of themselves, but they are vital for nutrients to be of use. To understand the relationship of enzymes to nutrients, consider what happens when building a house.

When a home is being constructed, various raw materials are brought to the construction site. One truck brings bricks; another unloads a pile a lumber. Screws, pipes, and coils of electrical wire are delivered. Plumbing fixtures, cabinets, and windows all lay around. All of these are raw materials delivered to the building site in the same way vitamins, minerals, and other nutrients are delivered to various sites in our body through the bloodstream or other route.

However, all those raw materials just lay there. They do not assemble themselves to construct the home. They do nothing. What is needed are the workers: the carpenters, the electricians, the plumbers, the masons. These workers come and pick up various raw materials and connect them together. They assemble and arrange the parts in the proper order. Carpenters pick up pieces of lumber, cut them into the right sizes, and connect them together. Electricians measure off wire and string it properly to make working circuits. Plumbers shape and organize pipes so water will flow in a certain direction. The workers also carry off the waste materials and debris, cleaning up the home for the new owners.

Enzymes are like the construction workers. They make things happen in biology. Enzymes handle the raw materials so the vitamins, minerals, and other nutrients can be of use. Without enzymes, the nutrients from our food and supplements just . . . do nothing.

On the other hand, enzymes are not vitamins or minerals. Taking enzyme supplements does not replace the need to have basic nutrition coming in as raw materials. You need to have good wholesome nutrients coming into the body, and then you need adequate enzymes to make use of those nutrients. They both work together.

It is important to remember that enzymes can only work with the nutrition that is in the food or supplements you are consuming. Enzymes cannot create a nutrient where there is none. No matter how many enzymes you dump on a cupcake, it just isn't going to magically transform into a healthy green salad.

Co-enzymes: Way to go, Partner!

Have you ever noticed how doing something with a buddy can just make a job go faster? At times, the results are much greater than simply multiplying by 2. Many enzymes have buddies that enhance their effectiveness. Often these assistants, known as co-enzymes, are required to enable the enzyme to work at all.

Co-enzymes are assisting compounds that bind to some part of the enzyme to significantly boost the enzyme's activity. Sometimes the binding changes the enzyme's shape so it can function. When the assisting compound is organic, like vitamin B12, it is called a co-enzyme. When the compound is non-organic, such as the mineral zinc, it is called a co-factor.

One of the most essential enzyme co-factors is the mineral magnesium. Around 300 enzyme reactions require magnesium.

Magnesium reactions promote good sleep, carbohydrate metabolism, calcium absorption, and proper nerve function. A deficiency in magnesium means compromising many necessary enzyme reactions.

Another common co-factor is the mineral zinc. Zinc is known for promoting a healthy immune system, reducing leaky gut (aids mucosal lining integrity), and keeping harmful bacteria in check. Zinc also is essential for an enzyme in the gut lining that is responsible for grabbing harmful heavy metals and removing them. Without zinc, this detoxifying enzyme activity cannot function (*see Chapter 2*).

This is the reason some enzyme products include small amounts of minerals. If sufficient co-factors are not present, you may not get the results you were hoping for from your enzyme supplement. Vitamins and minerals work together with enzymes, each acting as a key partner to get the entire job done.

Enzyme specialization

An important characteristic of enzymes is that they are highly specialized. Each enzyme has a certain 'job' that it does, and it does only that job. Just like a carpenter would not connect wiring. You would need an electrician to do that. Nor would the bricklayer install plumbing. Just as each construction worker is very skilled in his own area, each enzyme is very efficient at a single operation. Enzyme activities are not interchangeable, just like construction skills are not interchangeable. You will not have an enzyme which breaks down fats going up to help with respiration. Nor will an enzyme that works on dairy abruptly stop working on milk and go help the legs build muscle tissue. Not going to happen.

This high degree of specialization also contributes to enzymes being very safe. Enzymes do not wander around the body doing unexpected things, which is often the reason medications or other supplements create unwanted side-effects.

This very specific degree of specialization means that certain enzymes will be particularly effective for specific uses. Getting an appropriate enzyme or enzyme blend to break down a certain food, or to meet a particular health goal, is critical to seeing success with enzyme therapy. If you try an enzyme product and do not see the results you were hoping for, it could be the product is not designed for that specific use. Much like hiring a carpenter to wire your house. You very likely are not going to be happy with the results even if he does attempt the job. He might be a perfectly great carpenter, but he simply does not have the skills to do the job you want.

Fortunately, while this does present a little bit of a learning curve in the beginning, many enzymes products try to account for this. Companies will try to blend different enzymes together in one product so that all the different enzymes needed to accomplish a certain goal are included in the blend. This is why you will see a variety of enzyme products, some with very specialized target uses.

The art of enzyme blending

It is said that formulating enzymes is as much an art as a science. The science says that each enzyme has a certain type of job. Some of these jobs are quite specific while others are broader. For example, a protease is an enzyme that breaks down proteins. But there are thousands of different proteins and thousands of different proteases. Some protease enzymes only work on one type of protein bond that is quite specific.

One such case is an enzyme that only breaks a bond between a proline amino acid and a tryptophan amino acid. Another protease may break a more general type of bond. For example, it will break any bond where two of the same amino acids are connected together: two prolines connected together, two serines, two trytophans, two histidines, etc. Even though this second protease also has a specific action, it can actually be breaking a wider range of bonds than the first protease.

Consider a carpenter from our construction example. In the general sense, a carpenter works with wood, as opposed to an electrician or bricklayer. The general skill of 'carpenter' tells us it is someone who works with wood. This is like the general category of 'protease' which tells us it is an enzyme that works on proteins.

Now, different carpenters can have different specializations. For example, one carpenter may be able to frame the house, put up studs for the walls, assemble the rafters, and other broad-range tasks. But another carpenter may be called in to do fine custom detailing work on the mantel over the fireplace. Or another carpenter may make furniture and not work on home construction at all.

The fellow who works on furniture may have some limited ability to frame a house, and the guy who does detailing work may be able to crank out a coffee table, but neither would be as proficient in this side-area as they are in their area of specialization.

Enzymes operate in the same way . . . not that proteases can make furniture . . . but that they can have key areas of specialization, and yet may have some ability to work in another capacity, but just not as effectively. The important thing is not to stress out worrying that you have to learn about a zillion enzymes. Just keep this characteristic of specialization in mind when it comes to certain enzymes being needed for certain goals. It also comes up when trying to figure out why one blend of enzymes may work the same as another blend even if the ingredients are not identical. Similarly, you may have two products that look nearly identical and yet get very different results.

Let's look at how a blend of several enzymes mixed together has the ability to break more bonds than a single enzyme. Let's say we have a food with a basic structure as follows where the letters represent various amino acids:

A-A-A-A-B-B-C-C-A-A-A-A-B-B-C-C-
A-A-A-A-B-B-C-C-A-A-A-A-B-B-C-C

Enzyme 1 - breaks one specific bond

Now we add an enzyme that only breaks the bond between the structure B–C (B bonded to C). If we take this enzyme, the food will be broken this way with every bond between a B and C eliminated:

A-A-A-A-B-B   C-C-A-A-A-A-B-B
C-C-A-A-A-A-B-B   C-C-A-A-A-A-B-B   C-C

Even if we take vast quantities of this single enzyme, it will still only break that one type of bond. Food or substance breakdown will not exceed this degree of digestion.

Enzyme 2 - breaks a different and broader type of bond

If we add in another enzyme that only breaks duplicate type bonds (it breaks any bond between two similar amino acids), the food will be further broken down and look something like this:

A A A A-B B C C-A A A A-B B
C C-A A A A-B B C C-A A A A-B B C C

This enzyme has a slightly wider range in the types of bonds it will break than the first more specific one. It breaks bonds between two As, two Bs, two Cs, or any other duplicates whereas the enzyme in the first situation only broke one specific type of bond.

If we add both enzymes together in the same blend, we get far more complete breakdown than either enzyme alone.

The principle of combining enzymes, or blending, is a fundamental aspect of developing enzyme formulations. One very specific example is demonstrated by the enzyme company Enzymedica who has developed their own special process for blending. Each mix produced from this method is called a Thera-blend. Each Thera-blend represents a combination of similar types of enzymes that are selected for their ability to work together synergistically to more thoroughly break down a complex compound.

For example, in the protease Thera-blend there are actually three proteases selected for their ability to break down numerous bonds in a protein in different pH ranges. This effort requires more expense and skill to do; however, the goal is to develop a mix that is more efficient and effective at accomplishing a particular digestion goal. Because the blend is more efficient, you may need less actual quantity of a well-designed blend.

A practical example of this plays out in real life as a general principle when designing enzyme products to break down casein and gluten. Casein is a type of protein found in dairy, and gluten is a protein found in small grain cereals such as wheat, barley, and rye. Both proteins have a particularly hard-to-break, or digest, structure in one place. Research shows a certain enzyme activity known as DPP IV is needed to break a specific internal bond.

However, DPP IV alone will not break down the entire protein structure. DPP IV acts on a bond inside the protein structure. Two other general classes of protease enzymes are necessary to break down the outer protein structure so the DPP IV can gain access to the internal bond and work.

So, an enzyme blend targeting thorough casein or gluten digestion needs to have all three protease enzymes to be effective. There are several enzyme products effective for casein and gluten digestion currently available from various manufacturers using this blending format. Enzymes for gluten are discussed more in the next chapter.

Enzymes may be selected for other characteristics besides more complete breakdown a complex substance based. For example, in the Thera-blends, enzymes are chosen for their activity under a range of pH levels. pH changes throughout the digestive tract, so the idea is to maximize digestive action throughout the gut. Another enzyme formulator may be interested in other characteristics.

Plant- and microbial-derived enzymes are active and stable under a much wider range of pH levels and temperatures than animal-derived enzymes. The pH range of plant- and microbial-derived enzymes is generally said to be from pH 2 through pH 12. However, not every individual enzyme is optimally active in the complete pH range from 2 to 12. One enyzme may function from pH 2 to 6, another from pH 5 through 10, and a third from pH 4 to 12. In addition, although each enzyme has some activity in a given pH or temperature range, it will have a maximum activity somewhere within that range and lesser activity somewhere else.

Some enzyme makers specifically combine enzymes with this in mind. By combining enzymes with different pH ranges in one blend, a product is able to achieve greater enzyme activity over a broader pH range. This enables an enzyme formulation to break down more foods more thoroughly as the food and enzymes pass through the different pHs found throughout the digestive tract.

You could have a higher quantity of a single protease but this individual protease may be active in a narrower pH range and break a more limited number of bonds.

How can enzymes help

The 90 to 93% success rate observed with good quality enzymes is very significant (rates derived from studying hundreds of families over the course of several years; *Enzymes for Autism/Digestive Health*). This starts to make sense when you consider everyone needs to digest their food, no matter what eating plan they follow. Another reason the success rate is so high may be due to the fact digestive enzymes tackle problems on several fronts. Enzymes are probably one of the most basic and fundamental supplements to give. You get a lot of bang for your buck, so to speak.

1. Enzymes break down food particles so they do not exist as larger pieces which could physically irritate the gut lining or activate the immune system. Anything that does 'leak' through an injured gut lining while it is healing is less likely to provoke a negative reaction.

2. Enzymes release the individual vitamins, minerals, and other nutrients in food so the body can use them as the raw materials it needs. Enzymes also release the energy contained within food.

3. Enzymes allow you to get more nutrition from your food, even putting more whole-foods in the diet. You often do not have to supplement extra vitamins, minerals, and other supplements to compensate for what you eliminated through diet.

4. Enzymes work on the foods you do suspect as well as those you do not, or unknown sources. Food intolerances usually decline dramatically when using enzymes.

5. Enzymes proactively support intestinal health. They can act as trash collectors removing dead tissue, debris, chemicals, and toxins from the body. This cleaning out allows the gut to heal faster.

6. Another bonus is that enzymes are effective at clearing out pathogens that may cause and contribute to damaging the gastrointestinal tract. Bacteria, parasites, yeast, and viruses consist of organic compounds. Enzymes can help break these intruders down, and then carry off the toxins and dead cells the destroyed pathogens leave behind. Enzymes also work directly with the immune system to help control pathogens.

The many ways enzymes benefit health

Improvements with enzymes may be because enzymes work on many levels at the same time - different individuals benefiting for different reasons. Scientific evidence shows enzymes are effective in the following areas:

- Improve leaky gut
- Facilitate healing from disease
- Improve immune / autoimmune conditions
- Facilitate pathogen control
- Reduce inflammation and pain
- Faciliate detoxification
- Reduce or alleviate nutrient deficiencies / malabsorbtion
- Improve digestive function

---

7. Digestive enzymes themselves can be absorbed into the bloodstream. Along with other things, these enzymes, especially the proteases that break down proteins, can travel through the bloodstream cleaning out any gunk, toxins, and waste accumulating there. This assistance in cleaning the blood helps relieve the burden on the liver and the immune system. In addition, enzymes can work directly with the immune system increasing its natural effectiveness. Improvement in a variety of autoimmune conditions is associated with enzyme therapy.

8. Material leaking through the intestinal lining can make its way to joints and aggravate them to the point of inflammation, or add to existing inflammation. Proteases can reduce inflammation throughout the body, and thereby reduce many types of pain.

9. Because enzymes can work on a variety of problems at the same time and at the root level, some problems you may not even be aware of, you get a good value from your enzyme supplement investment.

Industrial uses - Are you wearing digestive enzymes?

Digestive enzymes have many industrial uses. All are based on their fundamental ability to break down specific compounds. Digestive enzymes may be closer to your heart than you realize. You don't really think those beloved stone-washed jeans were created by a bunch of employees huddled over a stream rubbing the denim down on some rocks?! Digestive enzymes are used to produce the many shades and textures of denim we so adore.

Manufacturers use digestive enzymes to treat and prepare a wide variety of fabrics. Different enzyme treatment processes give a fabric different looks, feels, drapes, strengths, and handling characteristics.

Cotton fabrics are treated with cellulase enzymes to permanently prevent pilling and 'fuzzing.' The enzyme process gives cotton more smoothness and softness, and a brighter, cleaner look. Amylase is used to desize material (a process of cleaning and softening fabric). Lipase works on oils in the preparation of leather.

Wool and silk are natural fibers containing proteins. These materials are often treated with protease enzymes to prepare the fabric, add the softness and lush feeling, and remove any impurities or roughness. Enzymes can make material easier to care for, including being machine-washable. Linen, hemp, and ramie processing involves enzymes as well.

Some fabrics actually rely on enzymes for their existence. Rayon is a man-made fiber made of regenerated cellulose derived from wood pulp or cotton linters. Cellulases are a big part in creating these fabrics. Variations of this process produce the materials viscose, cuprammonium, moldel, zantral, avril and lyocell (Tencel).

Enzymes are a great tool in fabric production. Enzymes are versatile, 'all-natural,' efficient, better for the environment, and replace harsh chemicals. They help protect our bodies both inside and out!

Other industrial uses of digestive enzymes include extensive use in the juice and baking industries. Enzymes are key in the manufacture of ethanol from plants such as sugar cane and corn. Digestive enzymes are fundamental in our world from making paper to processing plastics to cleaning up pollution. The number of industrial uses for enzymes is too extensive for this book. It is just interesting to know how ubiquitous and extensive enzymes are throughout nature and industry.

Breaking the barrier

I had to do something to that clay pan in the backyard if we were ever going to get grass cover. One way to help loosen up a clay soil is to increase the pH. Clay soils tend to be rather acidic with lower pHs, which limits nutrient availability. So I added lime to the area to raise the pH and improve the soil permeability. Over the next few months, I added thin layers of topsoil and compost to the area on top of the lime. The idea was to build up a good soil where there was none. The organic matter and minerals from the topsoil and compost layers would slowly trickle down mixing in with the clay layer being loosened up by the lime underneath. This would build a soil where grass roots could grow instead of the roots abruptly hitting a clay barrier. The growing roots burrowing down into the softening clay layer would help to disrupt it further.

All summer I layered on topsoil and compost every couple of weeks, and added a little more lime each month. The weathering process worked its magic throughout the fall and winter. The following spring I put down grass seed with another layer of soil and compost on top. The grass seeds appeared quite comfy in their customized soil. A lush grass sprung up on schedule burrowing down into the soil right away. Interestingly, we have not had any standing water in this spot since.

CHAPTER 4

Enzyme Nutrition

Technically, everyone and every living thing is always on a diet of some kind. A 'diet' is whatever eating plan you follow. It includes when you eat, the type of foods you eat, the types of food you do not eat, and any particulars involved in the eating, such as combining certain foods together, eating at certain times, or preparing foods a certain way. Even not eating can be considered a starvation diet.

People are individuals. Thus, different eating programs will be more or less beneficial to different people. What is 'the best' diet for one person may be radically different than the best diet for another. Peanut butter is a great source of protein and nutrition for many people, but must be banished for someone with a peanut allergy. Even choosing a diet that will be the most successful for weight loss will vary widely based on the person's lifestyle and metabolism.

Portion control

An important part of any diet is the concept of portion size. This is most important for weight control diets, but can affect the success of other diets as well. Be aware of not only what you eat but of how much you eat. Even with special diets promoting certain eating plans, most diets are designed to be followed in whole. If you pick out certain foods and eat large amounts of those, it could disrupt the original intention of the diet plan. For example, a low-carb diet may promote meats in quantity and low intake of carbohydrates. However, some people interpret that to mean they can gorge on baby-back ribs to their heart's desire and eat no carbohydrates at all. Then they are shocked when they are not losing the weight they planned on. The way they implemented the diet was never in the original plans of the diet designers.

Portion control and nutrient balance is a property of any healthy eating plan. Diets that stress specific types of fats or carbohydrates are not the same as a no-fat or no-carbohydrate diet. Nutrition works as a whole and is greater than the sum of its individual nutrient parts.

Nutrition and enzymes

Where do enzymes fit into diets and nutrition? The purpose and job of enzymes is to break down foods so the nutrition in the food can be used by the body. Without enzymes and the digestive process, how else will nutrients get into your body? You are not likely to get very far filling up your bathtub with nutritious food and soaking in it (although it might be an interesting experience).

Enzymes are the vehicle that facilitate getting the food you eat actually processed and into your body so the nutrients can do some good. Remember that just because you put something in your mouth and it disappears from view down your throat does not mean it is actually in your body. This applies to food, supplements, or medications.

When you put something in your mouth, which resembles a cave, it goes down the throat, a hollow tube. It passes into the cavernous stomach and eventually on through the nearly 26 feet of intestines, still a hollow tube. What is not absorbed continues out the other end. So essentially, we have a hollow core through our bodies.

Food, supplements, medications, and anything else remains 'outside' our body until it is absorbed across the intestinal lining and into our body structure. So, what you swallow is not really *in* your body until it is absorbed across the intestinal lining. Enzymes facilitate this process of getting what is flowing through the intestines broken down into a form that can be brought across the intestinal lining and into the body for use.

Think of nutrition as three basic parts:

1. Have adequate nutrition going into the body
2. Have adequate enzymes to release, absorb, and make use of those nutrients
3. Have adequate means to eliminate waste, residue, and toxins

The enzymes needed to release nutrients from food, supplements, or medications can come from the pancreas, the intestinal lining cells, saliva, in raw foods, or in supplements. Enzymes are destroyed by high temperatures or heat processing, so cooking deactivates any enzymes present in raw foods. There are some diets that actually emphasize enzyme rich foods as an essential component.

A main premise of raw food diets or 'juicing' is that you preserve and consume the enzymes which exist naturally in the raw food as well as the nutrients. Taking digestive enzyme supplements may achieve the same goal as it may not always be possible or desirable to do a 100% raw food diet.

Some diets promote the use of fermented foods: cultured vegetables, yogurt, kefir, and similar foods. The primary focus is to prepare foods so that they are a natural source of probiotics and enzymes in addition to the nutrients. Note that since probiotics produce digestive enzymes, anything with live probiotic cultures will also provide a natural source of enzymes. A diet including yogurt or other source of live probiotic cultures is a great way to keep your digestive health is good condition.

Enzymes consumed from food and through supplements can both be helpful in digesting food. However, there are some differences. On one hand, enzymes in a food source are working in a whole-food form, and they may be working more efficiently.

On the other hand, enzyme supplements can provide much higher concentrations than enzymes provided in food. In addition, supplements can allow you to select certain types of enzymes in various ratios. If you need higher concentrations of enzymes for therapeutic healing, supplements are necessary to supply these higher amounts. Taking enzymes as supplements in addition to food is another alternative to get the best of both sources.

Hey! What about the pancreas? Isn't the purpose of the pancreas to just crank out whatever enzymes you need? Why do we care if there are enzymes provided by food or in supplements?

The pancreas does respond to the food coming into the body, and does attempt to supply needed enzymes. However, to produce enzymes, your body uses raw materials and energy. These resources could be going toward other functions, like building muscle, providing stamina, fighting off disease, clearing out waste, and maintaining overall physical health. If energy and raw materials are excessively diverted to food digestion, overall health can suffer.

Supplying enzymes in food or supplements means the pancreas does not need to work as hard, and the body's resources can go into other functions. If you are ill, your body may desperately need these resources in order to heal faster. Some people have pancreas problems or serious digestive disorders. For these situations, supplemental enzymes may be necessary, and possibly lifesaving.

Supplemental enzymes also ensure food is more thoroughly digested. Poorly digested food can lead to numerous gastrointestinal problems including leaky gut, bacteria or yeast overgrowth that can feed on the undigested food, colon problems, more 'toxins' for your body to detox, a stressed immune system, digestive discomfort, and other maladies. Providing supplemental enzymes helps ensure this does not happen. And if you find you already suffer from one of these ailments, supplemental enzymes can help resolve the problem.

Nutrition from food versus nutrition from supplements

There can be a vast difference in results between nutrition from actual food versus taking synthetic supplements. Vitamins, minerals, and other factors work as a whole. Adding in or subtracting out selected components does not have the same biological value as the whole. This is the basis of 'whole-food' diets, or 'whole-food' supplements. In fact, taking larger quantities of synthetic nutrients over a long time may be detrimental to health.

Some studies point to the synthetics being treated as xenobiotic compounds by the body and excreted as such (meaning the body did not recognize it and treated it as a 'toxin'). One example is synthetic vitamin B6 which is commonly made from coal-tar (a phenolic compound). This is the same type of base used in artificial additives which can lead to a number of problems.

If you want or need to take a supplement, try to get one that is whole-food based or in the most natural form, when possible. Search online or ask in stores for 'whole-food supplements' or 'whole-food vitamins.' Be aware there are different views on this topic. When discussing 'synthetic vitamins' or looking at research, know that people may define 'synthetic' or 'natural' vitamins differently. Currently, all digestive enzymes are non-synthetic whether from an animal, plant, or microbial source. Advances in technology may provide other options in the future.

One of the big advantages of taking digestive enzymes is that it releases nutrition from food in a 'whole-food' form and allows the body to make maximum use of it. Enzymes not only prevent many of the problems created by poorly digested food, but also release the needed nutrition from food. You solve both issues at the same time. Of course, this is how our bodies were meant to operate all along.

Taking enzymes with nutritious food often brings much better results than using lots of synthetic supplements. This is very consistent with the results people using enzymes tend to see. Also, because nutrients in a whole-food form may be more efficient and effective, you may not need the same amount of a nutrient from a whole-food source compared to getting it from a supplement. Supplements are designed to s-u-p-p-l-e-m-e-n-t nutrition from whole-foods, not to be the staple form of nutrition in the diet.

That said, supplements can be very helpful in filling in nutritional gaps or correcting certain problems. Balance and a sensible approach are wise. I personally have had magnificent success using certain over-the-counter supplements used in certain ways for certain problems. Soluble magnesium has been great for my headaches, magnesium and zinc helped end one son's chronic chewing problems, and magnesium and probiotics helped our other son's bowel problems.

But there can be a scammish element to supplements because the supplement industry is not regulated. There are claims that some supplements can do everything for everyone - which is highly unbelievable. So caution is warranted. One should not throw away all their common sense or park their thinking skills at the door just because something is deemed 'alternative' or 'all-natural.'

Just because something is 'natural' does not mean it is safe used in any way you choose. Snake venom is 'all natural.' Hemlock is 'all natural.' Poisonous gases from the earth are 'all natural.' Use the same critical evaluation for all natural supplements as you would for any prescription medication or health therapy. If a medication or supplement is effective, it means it can cause a change in your body (hopefully for the better). So if it can effect a change, you need to make sure the change is managed properly so it goes in the appropriate way to the appropriate level. At a minimum, check for:

- How to properly use a new supplement or medication
- Maximum doses and how to dose
- Any interactions between supplements or medications

If you read all the literature and marketing brochures out there, you begin to wonder how you are able to stand up and breathe without a gallon of everything sold on the shelves! If you really tried to follow *all* the recommendations out there and take every supplement promoted, every day would be spent just taking supplements! There would be no room left for your life. There are so many health supplements that are allegedly good for our children and our selves, and so many diets claiming to be the best, how do you choose which one is the best?

When someone has impaired digestion for any reason (inflammation, yeast, bacteria, assorted toxins, poor diet, virus, surgery, metabolic problem, etc), a major issue is the lack of nutrient absorption across the board. And since any particular nutrient affects several areas in the body, if any one of them becomes deficient, multiple problems will then crop up in the body.

So with poor digestion or gut injury, *anything* you pull off the shelf in a supplement store has a chance of doing some good. That would explain why we hear improvements by a few people here or there associated with just about every nutrient known to man. This is also how people end up with long laundry lists of supplement upon supplement - 30, 40, or more a day. The pattern becomes giving the child or adult nutrition as individual supplements instead of through food. But nutrition does not really work very well via supplements alone. Science still does not understand nutrition well enough to manufacture the equivalent of whole-foods even if we had the capability.

In general, I feel the best approach to improve digestion and nutrition is to start with a good quality digestive enzyme first. This will help the body breakdown and absorb real food and get the best nutrition by that route. Then, after you start enzymes and get the child or adult eating the best whole-food diet they can tolerate, see what is left over in terms of symptoms needing correcting, supplements needed, or specific foods you still need to reduce or eliminate. It is very, *very* common that once a person starts enzymes, they find many foods can be added back to the diet. They also find many other supplements are not needed . . . or are not needed in as great a quantity.

The idea of supplementing is that supplements are in addition to a good whole-food rich diet, not instead of one. In fact, enzymes can make the supplements you do take much more effective. Anything you swallow, including special diet foods, medications, or supplements, still needs good digestion and absorption into the body to be as effective as possible.

From a very practical point of view, enzymes tend to be cheaper than many diets and excessive supplementation programs. From a gut healing point of view, stress itself can cause health problems and gut injury. You may be so stressed by trying to do a certain diet, or taking gobs of supplements, that you might not be gaining any ground in gut healing overall. If enzymes can help reduce that type of mega-stress on the family or child, that is just another positive benefit.

You can do a mix of enzymes, supplements, and food eliminations as well. It does not have to be all one or the other. Everyone has a different body and different situation. It is a matter of having options available so each person can find a workable solution for their situation.

Tip: A cheap and easy way to improve the digestion of food as well as digestive health overall is to *chew your food!* It's free! Chew, chew, chew. Try chewing each bite at least 20 times before swallowing. This will help develop the habit of more thorough chewing overall. The enzymes in your saliva will start mixing in with the food. Then in the stomach, the food particles have much greater surface area for the gastric acids and any enzymes present to work on.

Enzymes and special diets

Enzymes can be *very* effective in enhancing whatever diet you choose to, or need to, follow . . . even if it is no specific or special diet at all. Enzymes improve digestion and overall gut health. So whatever you eat, or whatever supplements or medications you take, they can be better absorbed and used by the body with enzymes. Supplements or food are not going to do any good just passing through the body.

Many diets are started because particular foods are not sufficiently digested, or cause digestion problems. Diets attempt to work around this by eliminating the problematic foods. However, a different more efficient strategy to consider is taking enzymes so the digestion problem is fixed at the core. Taking enzymes often can digest the foods in question such that the food no longer causes a problem. Thus, enzymes can make these food eliminations unnecessary. In addition, you then get your nutrition and energy from the food.

Whether or not enzymes can eliminate the need for a special diet depends entirely on:

- The enzyme product(s)
- The diet, and the goals or objective of the diet
- The individual's unique biology
- The person's lifestyle or situation
- Personal attitudes, beliefs, and preferences

Enzymes that are effective enough to replace special diets are a critical need for people unable to follow a diet 100% because of circumstances over which they have no control. Enzymes are also needed to help make a diet workable in everyday life. A situational need includes:

- If the person attends school, sleepovers, or other activities; there are other children not on the diet; a business dinner; or other situations where following or enforcing a diet is not possible

- If a child is in the care of someone who is not able to implement a diet, or does not want to follow a diet (ex-spouse, sitter, relatives)

- If there are situations beyond your total control (restaurant, traveling, product changes, hidden ingredients)

- If the stress of following a diet 100% just is not possible due to other situations in life (examples include a therapy, medication, job, or financial situation does not realistically permit meeting the demands of a rigorous or expensive diet)

Thus, enzymes can actually allow you to 'be on a diet' when it would be impossible otherwise. Some special diets are needed for medical reasons not focused on food breakdown. This is a separate issue from food eliminations based on the digestive process.

Example 1

A person may suffer a condition such as 'leaky gut' or bacteria/yeast problems. When there is substantial gut injury and digestion is compromised, *any food* eaten can become a problem. Any food insufficiently digested is a candidate to cross into the body or be absorbed when it should be screened out. This leads to food intolerance or allergy reactions to that food. This situation can develop into immune complexes, increasing toxin load, aggravating autoimmune conditions, and other unpleasant calamities. When this happens, everything starts to cause problems, and you start down a very slippery slope.

Let's say you think dairy and grains are a problem so you take those out of the diet. Maybe they are the foods you eat the most. You may even feel better. You start eating much more soy and corn as substitutes for the dairy and grains. Because digestion is still impaired, the soy and corn foods are now also insufficiently digested. They cross the injured gut lining and provoke the immune system to react. Slowly you develop food sensitivities to soy and corn. So then, you take the soy and corn out, and substitute in more, say, rice and fruits. But since digestion is still impaired, the same thing happens. Now these foods are poorly digested, and you may then develop sensitivities with these foods. You go through trying to eliminate food upon food until you have eliminated so many foods you turn around one day and find yourself on the food-free diet. You find you have become intolerant or sensitive to something like 27, 43, or 735 common foods. Taking something like a good broad-spectrum enzyme product to digest a wide range of foods is a basic start to get out of this cycle.

Example 2

Another example is a high protein/low carbohydrate diet. The objective here is to minimize carbs. Some diets focus on eliminating the type of carbs while others focus on the total quantity of carbohydrates. You might find taking an enzyme product specializing in targeting carbohydrates is not effective enough to replace the entire diet, but it does allow you to have more carbohydrates, both in type and quantity, than you could have otherwise. It may even eliminate the need for 50% of the diet restrictions, or 75%. Or perhaps you take it only with higher carbohydrate containing meals to help meet your diet goals. There are various scenarios possible with enzymes. Enzymes build in tremendous flexibility with diets which otherwise claim 100% strict round-the-clock compliance. This can substantially improve your quality of life as well as reduce costs for special diet foods.

Example 3

A third example would be the Feingold and Failsafe programs that eliminate certain artificial additives and possibly some naturally occuring food chemicals. One goal of the Feingold and Failsafe programs is to eliminate natural food chemicals (like salicylates, phenols, or amines) which may not be well tolerated. Enzymes may be able to break down foods in such a way the body is able to process these natural compounds appropriately without causing adverse reactions.

A different goal of Feingold and Failsafe programs is to eliminate synthetic additives. Since synthetic additives are not true organic food, enzymes are not very good at breaking these compounds down. Thus, enzymes may help with replacing the need for eliminating natural nutritious foods, but not the need for eliminating artificial chemicals. Artificial additives do not convey nutrition and can be detrimental to health over the long run so consuming them may not be wise whether you can stave off an immediate adverse reaction or not. Not surprisingly, digestive enzymes are phenomenal on food (that is the entire point of their existence after all) but not as effective on synthetic chemicals. Synthetic compounds are not 'food' per se so our bodies do not recognize them as nutrition for use. These ingredients tend to clutter up and add to the toxin load in our systems.

Example 4

Enzymes designed for casein and gluten digestion are successfully used instead of a GFCF (casein-free, gluten-free) diet by most people if they want to or need to do that with specific enzymes. Some people may prefer to eliminate foods because they just feel better about it. Some may want to use enzymes part of the time, but diet other times. Or another person may find enzymes work splendidly with casein but not 100% with gluten. Or they work with cheeses but not with milk because of a lactose intolerance issue (you would need the enzyme lactase for lactose intolerance). Most people find that adding enzymes greatly improves the results of the diet over just doing the diet alone. Some people find that enzymes for casein and gluten replace a GFCF diet with better results that even being GFCF with enzymes (that is, eating casein and gluten foods with enzymes gives substantially better results that being GFCF plus enzymes - this happens many times particularly in children with autism conditions).

Example 5

Athletes are often interested in maximizing protein intake. Not just intake, but actually getting their food and supplements converted into usable energy and muscle. In this case, you would not take enzymes with the goal of replacing a high protein diet and supplements. You would take enzymes to ensure that your food or supplements were maximally broken down, absorbed, and metabolized in the body. For proteins, you would consider something containing substantial protease.

Enzymes for gluten?

Gluten is a type of protein in certain cereal grains - wheat, barley, and rye - the basis of breads, baked goods, and pasta. The inability to sufficiently digest this gluten protein can lead to all sorts of symptoms including skin rashes, irritability, aggression, moodiness, 'brain fog,' cognitive problems, cramping, bowel problems, pain, and sleep disturbances. Avoiding gluten is very challenging as it is often used in small amounts in many foods. Digestive enzymes have been used very successfully for gluten intolerance in recent years. While some people are able to completely leave a gluten-free diet with appropriate enzyme products, others find the addition of these enzymes improves the success of their special diet, increases the range of foods they can eat, and improves their quality of life. Enzymes provide a great safety net to catch unknown or unavoidable sources of gluten as well.

Research determined the rate limiting bond in the digestion of certain proteins found in gluten, casein (a protein in dairy), soy, and possibly other foods requires an enzyme activity known as DPP IV (dipeptidyl dipeptidase IV). This enzyme activity is located in human intestinal cells in the gut lining. If you have gut injury these damaged cells will be unable to supply the needed DPP IV activity. For sufficient casein or gluten protein digestion, DPP IV needs to be present along with two other general types of proteases. (Byun 2001)

Gluten also contains a carbohydrate portion, another factor to consider. Some people have difficulty digesting the carbohydrate part of gluten, not the protein part. If you are following a low carb diet, or a specific carbohydrate diet, this is an area of concern. Remember that a number of enzymes necessary to finish digesting complex carbohydrates are also located in the intestinal lining, along the membrane of the villi structures. Any injury to the gut lining will also result in the loss of these enzymes when the cells are damaged.

A person may be sensitive or intolerant to gluten due to many reasons, two of which may be lack of sufficient enzymes to break down the gluten protein or the gluten carbohydrates. Artificial additives or other ingredients in baked goods are among other possibilities.

Several enzyme products targeting gluten digestion are currently available. Can these enzymes replace a gluten-free diet? While many people can replace a gluten-free diet with specific enzyme products, it really depends on the person and individual situation. First, note that some enzyme products for gluten (and casein) are only designed to assist a gluten-free diet or for trace amounts of gluten. These are not designed to completely replace a gluten-free diet.

Other products that are designed to replace a gluten-free diet work wonderfully for many people allowing them to completely leave a gluten-free diet. However, some people may not be able to complete leave a gluten-free diet, or at least not initially until some gut healing has occurred. Some people may be able to leave a gluten-free diet with one enzyme product but not with another product, even if the products appear relatively similar. Some people use enzymes for gluten to get even better results from their gluten-free diet, and to help with the many sources of hidden gluten or trace contamination. Some use these enzymes to eat gluten food occassionally.

Using enzymes to leave a gluten-free diet is meant for gluten intolerance due to gut injury, but not for the case of celiac disease. Celiac is a serious autoimmune condition different from other types of gluten intolerance caused by gut injury. In celiac disease, gluten actively injures the gut tissue and intestinal cells. The damage to the gut cells means the intestinal enzymes are not available to sufficiently digest gluten and casein. With non-celiac gluten intolerance, gluten is not the initial and main cause of the gut injury with the resulting loss of the intestinal enzymes. Any number of other things may cause the initial gut injury. This is the common scenario with autism, carbohydrate intolerance, and most digestive disorders.

Someone with celiac disease must stay gluten-free even with enzymes. However, most people with celiac have found enzymes very beneficial for their overall digestive health and for eating other foods. Many people with celiac find enzymes for gluten (and casein) allow them to have dairy, and help with accidental trace contamination. There is much ongoing research working towards developing an enzyme product or other supplement specifically for the celiac-gluten issue.

For specific enzyme products, trends, and possibly leaving or replacing a gluten-free (and casein-free diet), see page 108, *Special Note for GFCF diets (casein-free/gluten-free)* of the The Great Low-n-Slow Method.

Finding a qualified dietician or nutrition specialist

Enzymes are part of a total nutrition and digestive health program. The American Dietetic Association (ADA) has a great resource for finding a nutrition professional in your local area. You can visit the ADA website and type in a zip code to find a specialist in that area at: www.eatright.org. When contacting any specialist, ask about their area of specialization to see if it may be right for your situation.

Food for energy

When an enzyme breaks down food, not only are the nutrients in the food released, the energy that was in the chemical bond is also released. In animal science, energy is always a factor - a critical factor that goes into all feed calculations. In agriculture, the efficient conversion of energy and nutrients from feed to animal is a primary concern as a matter of business. Any feed expelled or not optimized by the animal is, literally, money down the drain.

I have noticed energy appears to be a lost variable in human nutrition. It is like trying to make the equation $a + b + c = ?$ balance without variable 'c.' What happened to the energy factor?

To understand where the energy in the food bond comes from, think of shaking hands with someone. When you grip the other person's hand, you need to put some energy into your grip in order to firmly hold onto the other hand. This is like a bond in food. When you let go of your grip, you relax your hand and the energy you were applying is now released.

It is common to hear that a child who was listless and sullen is now active and 'with it' after starting enzymes. Another common result with enzymes is an adult has soooo much more energy now! The fatigue is gone. The person feels so much better.

This may also be why some kids seem 'hyper' in the first days or weeks after starting enzymes. The child is getting a boost in energy from the food bonds being broken. After a few days or weeks, the person adjusts to the new influx of energy and it does not feel so odd.

When I first started taking digestive enzymes, I had a great deal more energy. Not hyperness, just more awake and alert. Like I finally got a really good night's sleep and had lots of spark. However, I was not used to this. I would sit around wide awake in the evening not really knowing what to do with myself. I was accustomed to being so fatigued by this point in the day I could barely stand. It took a good three weeks to fully adjust to feeling better. Even feeling better is a change. And change takes some adjustment until it is not so new.

The body can use the energy it gets from food for maintenance purposes or for growth. Maintenance include replacing blood cells, repairing muscle tissue, producing compounds needed for metabolism, removing by-products produced as a natural part of metabolism, and other aspects of keeping the body in good shape.

Growth includes adding on and expanding muscle tissue, bone cells, skin cells, brain neurons, and other body parts (not just replacing existing elements). Growth includes producing new compounds for the reproduction cycle or milk production in lactating animals. Growth usually happens after maintenance needs have been satisfied.

If the plant, animal, or person is ill, more energy needs to be diverted toward fighting off the disease. There is less energy for basic maintenance purposes and even less for growth.

Even if the objectives are not exactly the same, human nutrition can take advantage of all the research and information learned from animal science. Livestock producers are generally not concerned with whether their animals will grow up to attend college, marry well, and have a long fulfilling life. So at times, the model breaks down. However, animal science does allow experimentation and gathering information that would not otherwise be possible. This resource becomes invaluable particularly in the area of digestion and digestive health.

One area helping to bridge these differing objectives is pet nutrition. Pets are often cared for with the intention of having a long, pleasant life span. Interestingly, veterinarians often treat their animal patients for the same ailments as human doctors, particularly in the area of digestive problems. Enzymes are widely used in the area of veterinary medicine.

Realizing how essential the energy factor is in animal nutrition can go a long way in dealing with the effects seen in diet and enzyme supplementation. Often a person will start enzyme supplements and report something which could be related to an increase in energy levels. However, since they are not used to thinking about energy as a factor of nutrition, it can cause some confusion in what they are seeing or feeling. Most adults recognize when they have more energy even if they are not sure what is causing it. An adult may say they have less fatigue, less brain fog, or more energy.

With children, you are observing their behavior. The energy factor may not be as clear. It may be expressed something like the following:

"My son used to take a nap every afternoon and now he won't."

"My daughter doesn't want to go to sleep at her usual bedtime."

"My child wants to go outside and play now. He never wanted to do this before."

These reactions may reflect a burst of energy the child is getting from the enzymes breaking down more food. So it could be just having more available energy that the child is not accustomed to having. Feeling better is still feeling different!

The question I ask first when I get a concern like this is to ask how the child's disposition is. If the child is basically happy or pleasant, wants to play, is joking around, or needs more to do, this usually indicates they are adjusting to extra energy and could use more activity. Even if the child is on the hyper side, you can consider this as positive hyperactivity that soon goes away.

If the person is basically in a foul mood - picking fights, irritable, being destructive, etc. - this is generally not a feature of extra energy. It could be die-off from a pathogen problem, not tolerating something, or some type of adjustment to cleaning out the gut that is not related simply to an increase in energy. If the person is hyper in a destructive way, you can consider this as negative hyperactivity. There are several suggestions in the Troubleshooting section that may help with various causes of negative hyperactivity.

If you see a mixture of some improvements and some negatives, usually this indicates an adjustment is going on. The negatives usually fall away by the third to fourth week leaving only the improvements.

Nutrition over a barrel

An organic chemist named Justus von Liebig (1803-1873) is credited with devising the rate-limiting theory of nutrition, known as Liebig's Law of the Minimum. Developed for agricultural science, it has since been extended to applications in animal and human nutrition, as well as overall population dynamics. This Law states that overall growth is not controlled by the total quantity of all resources but by the amount of the scarcest needed resource. All the nutritional requirements of an organism need to be satisfied, or else the one in shortest supply will be the main cause for limiting growth. At one point, zinc may be the nutritional element limiting growth, then later it might be magnesium, and then later a vitamin or other nutrient.

Think of a barrel constructed with staves of different heights. Each stave represents a single nutrient or nutritional element. Some staves are short, representing a nutrient in short supply, while others are longer, representing a nutrient in greater supply. A thinner stave can represent a nutrient needed in less total quantity, such as a trace mineral, while a wider stave indicates a nutrient needed in greater total amount. Note that the amount of each nutrient required is relative to the organism's need. A trace nutrient may be present in small quantity, but this small amount may be sufficient to meet the overall need.

You can fill the barrel with water and it can 'hold water' (that is, growth will proceed) until the water gets to the level of the lowest stave. At that point, the barrel cannot hold any more water because the liquid sloshes out over the shortest slat. This shortest board is now limiting the rate of further growth. You need to increase the height of the lowest stave. Then you can add in more water until the water level reaches the next lowest board, which then becomes the element limiting growth. Even the very narrow short stave of a trace nutrient will let out the water and limit growth should it become insufficient. (Purdue University 2005; The Fertilizer Handbook 1982)

This is why mega-dosing nutrients may not be the best route in supplementation. If the rate-limiting nutrient is, say, vitamin B12 and you supplement B12, you may see an increase in growth initially. The

Liebig's Law of the Minimum

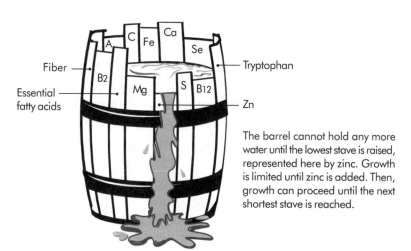

The barrel cannot hold any more water until the lowest stave is raised, represented here by zinc. Growth is limited until zinc is added. Then, growth can proceed until the next shortest stave is reached.

addition of B12 increases growth until another nutrient then becomes the nutrient in shortest supply and cannot meet the overall need. Maybe the rate-limiting nutrient then becomes zinc. Adding more B12 at this point will not increase growth now. Additional zinc is what is needed to overcome the growth limitation. This does not mean it was a mistake to go with B12 and not zinc in the beginning. Zinc was not the nutrient limiting growth the most at that particular time. Keeping an eye on balance in nutrition is key to overall health and healing.

There is also an unofficial Law of the Maximum where you may reach an upper limit of a nutrient. Some nutrients actually cause problems in higher amounts and can even reach toxic levels. When considering any nutrient, look at both the minimum and maximum levels to see if high doses are a cause for concern.

To add to the complexity, as the organism grows, or heals, the nutritional needs shift. All this helps explain why you may find yourself constantly adjusting and re-adjusting a nutritional program, especially while trying to overcome a chronic health issue. Knowing this lets me know I am not doing anything 'wrong' if I find I need to make changes in a nutritional program every few months. It is all part of the process.

I like to know what to expect as much as possible. I was fairly sure of what to expect with the yard renovation, and how the process basically worked. I just 'expected' it to move along much more quickly. And when I started digestive enzyme therapy, I was fairly sure of how enzymes worked in general. However, I was not prepared for the lack of practical information on what to expect with digestive enzymes. The area was a huge blank. This was a bit frustrating as someone considering a new therapy for health, particularly when it is for your kids. What exactly were you getting into with this enzyme stuff? After quite a few years, a ton of effort, and lots of contributions volunteered from other regular families, trends in enzyme therapy emerged.

CHAPTER 5

Just for the Record
– Trends in Enzyme Therapy

It was the best of enzymes. It was the worst of enzymes. It was the season of improvements. It was the season of disappointments. It was the age of learning. It was the age of research. This is a tale of two enzymes. Well, actually a lot more than just two.

When I started investigating digestive enzymes for gut problems in humans, what struck me most was the complete lack of order and direction. It was chaotic at worse and just a huge blank unknown at best. There were no guidelines to help one get started with digestive enzymes, no outline for what possible reactions may mean, and no way for someone to tell if they were 'doing it right.' While there were loads of research studies showing enzymes can be effective, and many enzyme supplements on the market, there was no outline or guide that dealt with the practical application of enzyme therapy.

I like to know what I am getting into. As much as possible anyway. Knowing what to expect can go a long way towards a therapy being successful or not. For example, if you are aware that starting enzymes or probiotics may increase energy levels, you can prepare for being more awake or a bit of hyperness in your child. However, if you are not aware this can happen, you could be surprised, alarmed, or confused at the reaction.

It is also helpful to know things such as 'will I need to take enzyme supplements the rest of my life?' This chapter outlines some of the general trends seen with digestive enzymes as compiled following thousands of cases of enzyme use since 2001. This discussion is intended to present a rough idea of what to expect when taking digestive enzymes to help you make better decisions. Please keep in mind each person is an individual and actual results may vary.

I have been tracking trends since 2001 and with thousands of cases. The information collected would not have been possible if not for the gracious efforts of many individuals taking the time to monitor their own personal results and share them with others. Thanks to all these anonymous contributors for their volunteer efforts.

Great expectations

Here is a list summarizing common improvements seen with good quality digestive enzymes. You may see different improvements depending on what the starting problems were. Note also that benefits with enzymes may appear as negative things that no longer happen. A child may simply not be as fussy anymore, or an adult finds they have more energy and can complete tasks they would get too tired to accomplish before.

Sometimes the improvements are very drastic from the very beginning, even the first day, while in other cases the benefits slowly increase over time. Notice that some of the improvements relate to physical changes (such as better bowel regularity or improved sleep) while others reflect improvements in behavior. Each of these improvements was discussed in detail in my previous enzyme books *Enzymes for Autism/Digestive Health.*

The good stuff - Possible improvements where there were problems

- Increased bacteria, yeast, and viral control, less illness
- Increased energy, decreased fatigue
- Decreased pain
- The Happy Child Effect (pleasant overall disposition)
- Increased eye contact and attention
- Increased language and communication

- Improved sleep
- Increased number of foods tolerated (physically)
- Increased foods accepted by choice (preference)
- Gained weight, if needed
- Lost weight, if needed, and reduction in cravings
- Improved stools/bowels regularity
- Improved skin color and overall appearance
- Improved transitioning and flexibility in routine
- Increased desire for physical activity
- Decreased general anxiety
- Improvement in socialization, humor, affection
- Increased awareness, less 'brain fog'
- Increased problem solving and cognitive ability
- Improved short-term memory
- Increased range of interests
- Increased light, sound, and color tolerance
- Improvement in other sensory issues
- Decreased aggression, moodiness, anxiety
- Decreased hyperness, aggitation
- Decreased inappropriate repetitive behaviors
- Decreased self-injurious behavior
- Decreased required medications and supplements

At times, improvements may not seem very related to initiating use of enzymes. For example, several times a parent wrote the child started enzymes and began to go outside and play on the swing-set whereas before the child was frightened of playground equipment and refused to go near it. While on the surface it may look as though playing on a swing-set has nothing to do with taking enzymes, closer inspection can reveal the connection, providing a logical explanation.

I suffered chronic migraines for years. A common effect of migraines is distortions in vision, a feature I apparently was graced with as well. I say 'apparently' because I was not really aware of the degree of the problem until it stopped. There are different types of migraines. The type I had did not come and go throughout the months. The type I had came when I was about 11 years old, stayed, and took up residence for the next few decades. It was a constant round-the-clock thing day after day, month after month.

When I started a medication for migraines, and further when I started enzymes, the migraines pain went away. A 'side-effect' was that my vision apparently corrected, most notably in the area of depth perception. Apparently, I had gotten so used to functioning with the distorted vision, I did not realize it was 'off.' When it was corrected, it took some getting used to; very similar to living with poor eyesight and then getting brand new glasses. Yes, you see better, but it is still different and takes some getting used to.

In my case, I noticed this adjustment most when going up and down stairs. I tended to overshoot the distance just slightly when putting my foot down. When getting a drink, I would tip the glass a bit as I misjudged the distance. After a few weeks, all of this went away, just as one adjusts to new eye glasses or contact lenses.

My older son also had this problem with judging depth perception. It also went away when he started a medication for migraines and with enzymes. Even as a toddler, he would get positively hysterical if he needed to walk on stairs without risers or had openings in the slats (when the steps were not completely closed and you could see some of the ground through the steps). He would get frantic if there was a grate in the sidewalk, and walk way around it. He would also avoid swings, slides, and other typical playground equipment because of the depth perception problem. Correcting the visual disturbances made these behaviors go away. He 'suddenly' started playing on the playground with the other kids.

Migraines and head pain can be caused by food intolerances. If enzymes can break down a problematic food so it does not cause these head problems, the behaviors resulting from the head pain would disappear as well.

This example is just one of many that have come up over the years. The point is you may see all sorts of changes that initially seem totally unrelated to enzymes or digestion when starting enzymes. Enzymes work on many aspects of health all at the same time that can lead to a very wide variety of possible improvements.

How we talk about health: adults versus children

The same physical things may be happening to children as they do adults. Digestion works the same in both groups. However, we tend to talk about health differently depending on whether the person is a child or an adult.

With children, we generally discuss health in terms of behavior. Describing a child's behavior is meant to tell us something about their state of health:
- "Emma must not be feeling well. She sat on the side as the other children played at recess"
- "Mark fussed all during lunch. He only ate a few chips."
- "He was much better today. He went out to play on the swings."

Children are unable to express how they feel as adults can. My preschooler is not going to come up and say "Mommy, I have a migraine with visual distortions and nausea." He will just know he feels badly, act out, and might even start banging his head on the ground to get some relief from the pain.

With adults, we generally talk about health in terms of productivity. Describing how much work an adult gets done is supposed to tell us something about their state of health or how well they are feeling:
- "Amy was so sick she left work early and went home." The fact Amy was no longer able to stay at work is supposed to convey some sense of how ill she is.
- "How is John doing? That was a bad accident he was in." "Oh, much better. He will even be back at work next week." "Wow, that's great. I'm glad he is recovering so quickly."
- "I was feeling better so I mowed the lawn and mulched the shrubs this weekend."

Just remember the same things may be going on healthwise with both children and adults, but we tend to talk about them differently. Digestive enzymes may produce similar results in both groups, but the language used to describe the situation may be different.

The not-so-good stuff - Possible adjustment reactions

Likewise, changes can be . . . unsettling. When introducing something that causes change, even when the changes are working towards improving health, there can be some uncomfortable symptoms as the body adjusts. Most of these adjustment effects end by the third to fourth week. Most people say the adjustments are quite manageable and not too disruptive. However, at times the adjustments can be more severe, particularly if you start enzymes at an aggressive dose or have a very sensitive gastrointestinal system. This may be referred to as a 'healing crises' - part of the initial process of the body healing.

The symptoms you may see are referred to as adjustment effects instead of side-effects. Side-effects typically refer to symptoms that occur as long as you pursue the particular therapy or product. For example, a side-effect of a medication may be you get dry mouth. As long as you take the medicine, you experience a dry mouth. If you are taking the medicine 20 years from now, it continues to cause dry mouth. It is a constant effect of taking the medication.

Adjustment effects from enzymes are different because they happen while the body is adjusting to the change. After a few days to a few weeks, once the body adjusts, the symptoms go away. The general guideline is that enzymes should be tried for at least three to four weeks to allow for common adjustments. Most of the adjustment effects result from:

• The body processing more food and liquid
• Gut healing, cleaning out debris, reducing inflammation
• Die-off from yeast, bacteria, or other pathogens in the gut
• Withdrawal effects from 'addictive' food compounds
• The body receiving more nutrition from food or supplements

Hyperactivity, irritability, withdrawal, or allergy-like symptoms can actually be indications the enzymes are working and the body is adjusting. The most common adjustments to enzyme therapy are discussed in detail in the enzyme books *Enzymes for Autism/Digestive Health* and at www.enzymestuff.com. They include temporary hyperactivity (various reasons for this), stomach ache, thirst, or changes in stools. Please note that many people do not experience any uncomfortable adjustments at all. If you see only improvements, do not think you are doing something wrong.

The development of The Great Low-n-Slow Method for beginning enzymes has vastly reduced the uncomfortable adjustment symptoms some people experience. This method is discussed in the next chapter and is highly recommended for children, those with serious digestive injury, or those with sensitive systems.

Additional trends

The following trends have remained very consistent over the years, and occur with good quality appropriate enzymes from various manufacturers.

- 90 to 93% of people using an appropriate good quality therapeutic enzyme product see at least some improvement. This varies between small yet noticeable improvements to large sudden improvements in health and behavior.

- Usually you can tell if enzymes are working in three to four weeks, or one bottle of enzymes. For older kids, teens, and adults, you may need to allow a little longer - around six to eight weeks instead. See the following section on older children and adults for details. Even if there are uncomfortable or questionable reactions, you can usually tell that something is happening anywhere from the first day to several weeks. The basic investment is one or two bottles of enzymes and around to four to six weeks. We are not talking about spending months or hundreds of dollars trying something before being able to determine if it helps.

- Besides food breakdown, certain enzymes can help with gut healing, controlling pathogens, and immune system support. The general trend is most people do see improvements in these other health related areas besides food digestion even if they are only taking enzymes for food digestion. A nice side-effect!

• Most people say taking enzymes does help reduce the cost of their health program overall as well as saves time and effort.

• Generally, the longer you take enzymes, the less enzymes you need for the same results, not more. This is probably the result of gut healing and overall improvement in health. As your own digestive system improves, your body's enzymes may be functioning better, even improving your own body's enzyme production. When the intestinal cells are damaged, the enzymes produced by the intestinal cells will not be available. Taking digestive enzyme supplements can help to heal the gut. As the intestinal cells grow again, the healthy new cells are then able to produce digestive enzymes.

• Some people find they get better results if they use enzymes with all meals and snacks, particularly in the beginning months. I found that in the beginning months I needed to give enzymes each time there was even a little bit of dairy in any meal or snack. After about the fifth month, I did not need to give enzymes with trace amounts of dairy and could even skip enzymes with a dairy-laden meal once every four days. By the ninth month, we could go several meals a week without enzymes. By the first eighteen months, enzymes were needed with dairy only half the time, and eventually enzymes were not needed at all.

• There is steady improvement the longer you continue enzymes. Any initial improvements do not 'wear off' and disappear; and further improvements generally appear after the initial few weeks.

• Initially, there was some concern that a person may develop an intolerance to enzyme supplements in the same way they develop sensitivities to foods and some other supplements. However, to this date, there have not been any reports of this happening.

• Enzymes usually allow you to add most of previously eliminated foods back into the diet. Some people can add back in all previously eliminated foods, but other people find they may still need to eliminate a couple foods or chemicals (such as artificial additives, amines, or highly phenolic foods).

- The vast majority of people adding enzymes to their special diet find the enzymes give them another jump in improvement.

- Results found with the previous Seven Month Study based on two enzyme products in particular have since been found and maintained with several different quality lines of enzymes. Further innovations in enzyme products have emerged as well providing even better results for various situations than before.

Older children and adults

Since the writing of the previous enzyme books, there is much more information on enzymes and older children and adults. An 'older' child refers to someone around age six and up. Older children through the age of ten to twelve, or up to puberty, are just as likely to show improvement with enzymes as younger children are. The improvements in older children tend to be just as significant and just as immediate as with younger children. This trend appears whether the child is on a restrictive diet or not.

For those individuals past puberty, the improvements may be as immediate and significant as with younger children. However, the degree of improvement may also be lower in the very beginning. There may also be a lag in improvement where you may need to allow around six to eight weeks to see improvements instead of the usual three to four weeks. Now, in the grand scheme of things, eight weeks is still relatively quick when discussing major changes in health. Good improvements do come for most older individuals.

One reason older children or adults may take longer to show improvement may simply be because they have had longer to incur more pronounced and extensive problems which take a little longer to correct. They have had more time to develop far more gut damage, food intolerances, and metabolic problems than younger children.

Another reason may be because older people have learned various coping skills and behavior patterns along the way. They may go through a period of adjusting to feeling better before their outward routines and behaviors change to something noticeably different. Feeling better is still feeling different.

Another trend that surfaced is older children and adults generally show greater positive results with enzymes than with restrictive diets alone. This includes both the case where enzymes are added to a restrictive diet, and when enzymes are used instead of food eliminations.

Eliminating any one or two foods (such as just gluten and casein) may simply not be enough to achieve the greater levels of improvement because an older child has had more time to develop more extensive gastrointestinal problems. Even if many foods are removed, food eliminations may not enhance gut healing.

Let's say a younger child has developed food intolerances to three different foods whereas an older child has progressed to developing food sensitivities to 17 foods. If the parent removes the four major foods she thinks are a problem, this may cover all of the younger child's issues, but would only account for a fraction of the older child's.

Using enzymes breaks down all foods at the same time. This means that both the younger child's three foods as well as the older person's 17 foods would be addressed. Thus, a broader range in age groups tends to show greater improvements immediately with enzymes.

Another factor contributing to why older children tend to see greater improvement with enzymes than on restrictive diets could be the care-giving environment. Parents and other caregivers have more absolute control over the diet and environment of younger children. Older children are more independent and have more opportunities for exposure to off-diet products making strict adherence to a diet difficult.

Parents of elementary school-age children trying both the enzymes and restrictive diets find their children are far more willing to comply with taking enzymes plus foods they enjoy than adhere to a strict diet. School-age children and teens tended to be surprisingly cooperative in taking enzymes, even reminding their parents and teachers. Older children may be better able to understand they just felt better taking enzymes. The main reasons given by children for preferring enzymes are wanting to participate in social activities, eating school lunches, feeling better, and just being able to eat something they preferred.

In situations where enzymes are given for autism, ADHD, and related conditions, socialization is a primary problem. Special diets tend to separate children out or isolate them from others and may create additional social hurdles. This only adds to the problem they are attempting to overcome. Enzymes can be a great solution for addressing their digestive needs without creating further problems with socialization.

Better bedroom behavior

Okay, this is the 'adult' section of the book, added in because of certain undeniable trends not addressed before in other books.

Over the years, both men and women have commented, usually very privately, that taking digestive enzymes enhanced their intimate relationships. Apparently, certain enzymes can result in adding more zest to sexual experiences. Various reasons may explain why this unexpected 'benefit' turns up.

Certain enzymes taken between meals promote improved blood and oxygen circulation (nattokinase, serratiopeptidase, and perhaps other proteases). Circulation problems have been an issue for some men in intimate relations. Improving circulation is a prime mode of action of several currently popular medications for erectile dysfunction. Improving blood flow and circulation through enzymes may contribute to the improvements seen in this area. Enzymes also have the direct effect of supplying more energy from food breakdown. Both increased energy and increased circulatory function can increase stamina and decrease overall fatigue.

Enzymes may simply be assisting in the area of intimate relations because they improve general health overall. When someone is ill, any activity can be difficult. In my case, I used to have such serious migraine pain, being around someone, anyone at all, took effort. When the migraines cleared up, any type of socialization was far easier. It is difficult for anyone with physical pain to engage in physical activities of any sort. As health improves, romantic activities tend to improve along with other physical activities.

In a related issue, a number of women have commented that beginning enzymes made their monthly periods regular when their cycle was quite irregular before. A few women conveyed they had never been regular until they started enzymes. Then their periods became regular, even at ages of 30 to 40 years old.

Women suffering from PMS say enzymes drastically reduced their PMS associated problems. The improvements seen include the number of problematic symptoms brought on by PMS, the intensity of the symptoms, and the duration the adverse symptoms lasted. Female issues included better regulation of monthly blood flow, less breast soreness, and reduction or elimination of cramping. Intense mood swings went away completely for some women while others said their problems were greatly reduced. A few women mentioned periodic spotting between cycles ceased.

At this point, I have not found research information specifically on whether enzymes help regulate hormone imbalances. However, some work is underway looking at enzymes and hormones in general.

Gender specific issues are an area of enzyme therapy that has not been widely investigated formally. However, if you start enzymes and notice significant improvements in areas of sexual health, know it is not just your imagination. There are logical explanations why you may be seeing benefits in these areas, and others are experiencing similar results.

Four possible reaction patterns

The four general patterns to look for when you start enzymes are as follows. First, you or your child may show only positive reactions when starting enzymes and no negatives at all. This is common. In this case, simply rejoice for the blessing of smooth sailing.

The second very common result when starting enzymes is to see a mixture of some positive improvements *along with* some unwanted adjustment effects. It is really important to notice if there are any positive improvements at all occurring at the same time you see some negatives.

An example would be if you see your child has stopped being such a picky eater, is much more 'with it,' and now sleeps much better. At the same time, the child may be a bit more whiny and refuse to clean-up their things where previously this was not a problem. A mixture of some positives along with some negatives usually indicates the person is going through the initial adjustment phase. After a few days or weeks, the negatives go away leaving only the positives.

Although most people do see some type of improvement with enzymes, some do not. About 5% see only negatives or no positive results, which is the third possibility. This is when you really need to keep your eye on things. Sometimes the cases showing only negatives are still cases of temporary adjustments where die-off from pathogens may be masking any improvements. But sometimes the initial all-negative reactions are related to an intolerance to the products used, or possibly an additive or filler in the product. A different product or therapy may be needed.

If you only see negative symptoms and no positive responses *at all* past the first three to four weeks, discontinue enzymes or consult your doctor, the manufacturer, or other people using enzymes (such as in the enzyme discussion group given in the reference section). Often these sources can review your situation and lend suggestions on what may be going on and what you might be able to adjust. People who participate in the discussion group or seeking advice tend to have significantly more positive results than those who do not. This is simply because of the assistance and sharing of experiences that can clarify or improve your enzyme program.

What if you do not see any change? Nothing positive or negative. A blank. Zip. Nothing at all. This is the fourth possibility: nothing positive and nothing negative. The first thing to try is to increase the dose of the enzymes or other pathogen control measures. It could be the enzymes are working but at a level that is so low and well tolerated you do not see any adjustment reactions, but yet it is not sufficient enough to produce visible improvements.

If increasing the dose sufficiently does not produce results, try a different enzyme product in the same category (such as 'yeast targeting', 'strong protease,' 'broad-spectrum,' etc.). Enzyme blends can have very different or specific overall actions even if the labels are fairly similar. One formulation may be much more effective for a particular individual than another blend. Try at least one other enzyme product in the same category before giving up. Most reputable supplement companies allow you to return opened but unfinished product, if you need that option.

Note: Check the Troubleshooting Guide for various reasons you may not see the results you were hoping for and suggestions to try.

For everything there is a season

Fortunately, time, effort, and research have paid off and now there are good guidelines for enzyme therapy. It is less chaotic than before, and more than the ocean of emptiness it once was. Finding new guidelines takes time. Sometimes it requires lots of thought, tedious plodding through published research, testing, evaluation, refining the idea, and then testing again. Other times interesting results just pop up by accident all on their own. And still with others, it takes some time to see how various approaches shake out in real life.

The improvements with enzymes my own family has seen took place over time. My older son had debilitating neurological problems since he was several weeks old. He was nine years old when we started enzymes and he responded wonderfully. We have used several brands and types of enzymes over the years for different issues. Of course, enzymes were not the only therapy we tried that helped, but it was a notable part. Over the many years, we also found success with sensory therapy, two medications, lots of one-on-one teaching, behavioral education, and lots of love among other things.

My younger son had serious gut problems since he was an infant as well: projectile vomiting, gagging reflex/GERD, bowel problems, encopresis, bacteria infections, and eventually he just stopped eating and growing. We burned through a multitude of doctors, each contributing what they could to these complex problems.

So how are the boys doing now? How are we faring after all these years? Quite well, overall. The improvements we saw with enzymes never left. In addition, old problematic coping behaviors have melted away. Younger Son's digestive problems and reflux are under control, with many of the problems fading over time.

My older son's chronic head-banging has been replaced by a persistent sense of humor and creative outlook. The nightmarish torrents of screaming a thing of the past.

Both boys have finished their black belt program in Taekwondo, and the oldest has taken a fancy to fencing. He took to the sword right away. Yep, that's my son. Give that boy a sharp, pointed object and he is good to go!

Trying new things used to be a huge problem for our older son. The slightest change in his pre-planned schedule could send him into a tailspin. There were so many times when he was young he would collapse into a blistering screaming fit of frustration if we veered off the planned route even a little. His hyper-sensitive sensory issues were just too intense for him to cope. But now, that is all a distant nightmare and he can transition relatively well, although he still prefers a little lead time to adjust. But that is typical of many people.

I plopped down on the couch next to Older Son, who was busy sketching one of his many heroic characters . . . his 'guys.'

"So, when do you want to go get our bricks?" I asked in the most upbeat way possible so as to make it seem like hauling heavy blocks of concrete to shore up a retaining wall was the most fun we could ever have.

Uh-oh! Matthew was on the alert. He smelled work. *Our* bricks? 'Our' means that *we* would be the ones getting the bricks. And since *I* am the young becoming-ever-so-handsome dashing dude out of the two of us sitting here, it is reasonable to think *I* would be the one lifting most of the bricks. Wait! What about that other brother? He's got to help too.

"Your brother is going, too," I added. I can read minds. "But you can choose when we go because he chose the last time."

"After college." Matthew said flatly, going back to his sketching. He hoped that maybe saying it with enough authority would somehow make it true. Matthew still didn't turn on a dime when it wasn't his idea to do so.

"'Fraid not. Choose a time between now and Friday." Giving him a choice has always worked before in smoothing over resistance. Matthew tended to bolt if he felt trapped into a situation. "If we get done early enough, we can stop by the bookstore and you guys can see if there is a new game magazine out," I offered.

Matthew took a shot at reasoning with me, "If I break my back moving those blocks around, my brother will have to waste all his money taking care of me forever. And when you are old, rusty and crusty in a nursing home, I won't come and feed you mashed potatoes."

I gazed at the ceiling casually, "The potatoes would probably be soggy anyway."

By now, Matthew had had enough time to mentally adjust to a change in his planned activities. "We can go after lunch. I'd rather get this over with. I want to read the new game reviews anyway and see if anything good is coming out 'cause I already beat my other games."

Yes, this was a vast improvement over the past.

I surveyed the improvement on the yard as we ended the summer season, now going into fall. Although there was progress, the improvements were not nearly as vast as I had hoped. On top of that, a few unexpected items were appearing. Like that sinkhole in back where the 30-foot trench was dug out. It started out as just a slight depression that I could convince myself was simply a trick of the sun's light. However (and you just knew there was going to be a 'however'), the ground sank more, then more. By fall, the hole was so pronounced we had to mow around it lest the mower fall in and get stuck.

And several very large bushes (small trees) were now dying where the trenching equipment had fatally damaged their root systems. Those would all need to be dug up and replaced. *Arrgggh!!!* That was soooo *not* in the plan! At least the grass cover seedlings were coming in fairly well. I was working with smaller more manageable patches, one area at a time. However, I was reluctantly having to accept that complete restoration would take several more seasons . . . a slow process but one that could bring permanent results.

CHAPTER 6

The Great Low-n-Slow Method

One thing is for sure; when you are waiting for the grass to grow . . . it's like . . . watching grass grow! Slow and steady. You can optimize the growing environment so conditions promote the most growth, but past a certain point, you simply cannot force it anymore. Trying to force growth too much can actually delay it.

Our younger son was in charge of watering several patches of grass seeds we were trying to establish to fill bare spots in the yard. These 'spots' covered several square yards each. We had already added topsoil and organic matter to enhance the growing environment. Younger Son was supposed to gently water several times a day for a couple weeks in order to keep the ground moist. If the ground dried out, it would hamper seedling growth. The process required a gentle yet steady input of water.

This nurturing process wasn't exactly a certain boy's style.

"Whoa! You can't dump water on like that!" I yelled rushing over and grabbing the hose from his hand. Instead of gentle rains, the gasping seedlings were being subjected to a typhoon as they were flooded with torrents of water at full force.

"Of course I can," the brown-haired boy said casually, rolling his eyes toward the sky, hoping that saying it out loud would somehow make it true. I shot him a glare while turning the water pressure down.

"Let me rephrase that: you can't flood the seedlings like that and expect them to live! Dumping tons of water or fertilizer on a plant will not hurry up the growth process."

Gently, I continued explaining, "As much as I would like to, it isn't possible to reach down into the earth and yank those seedlings up and out as flourishing full-grown plants. You need to go slower with lower amounts of food and water for the plants so they can actually make use of the nutrition without getting overwhelmed by it. Otherwise they get damaged. The problems slow down their growth. Just because a little of something is helpful does not mean more is better."

The young one frowned at the mention of fertilizer. The Fertilizer Incident, as it was now known, only happened because he was trying to be efficient. Efficient sounded better than lazy. Instead of spreading the fertilizer out loosely in thin, even layers, he attempted to save time by dumping it out in hefty handfuls. He figured it would all even itself out anyway on the ground.

It didn't. It ended up laying in clumps. This promptly burned all the little plants under the clumps, killing them out. The entire area that had just started to fill in with a layer of young grass had to be stripped out and the ground cleared of excess fertilizer salts. This delayed establishing the ground cover several weeks to say nothing of the additional labor. The chore was made more annoying since he had to endure the constant ranting from his brother about why they were having to redo the same area all over again.

Younger Son picked up a shovel and started pounding out loose dirt clods far more forcefully than necessary, taking his frustration out on the ground. Poor little dirt clods.

I handed him the hose back demonstrating a sweeping motion which allowed a fine mist of moisture to cover the seedlings. Then, said encouragingly, "Give it another go, why don't you. It takes time to get the hang of this, just like it takes time for the plants to grow. It's a process."

He smiled as the meaning registered in his head, "Just like when you tried to learn how to cook beef?"

I cringed at the mention of what is now affectionately referred to as The Great-Shoe-Leather-Saga.

"Yeah. Just like that."

Just as plant growth is a process, repairing injured tissue in the gut, or anywhere for that matter, takes a certain amount of time. Healing is a process. While we want healing to happen as quickly as possible, going too aggressively can cause problems of its own.

Enzymes have pro-active healing properties. While this is wonderful for health, experience has shown that going too aggressively can cause unwelcome discomfort for some people. Starting lower and slower tends to be particularly helpful in the beginning, especially for those with sensitive digestive or nervous systems, those with extensive gut injury, or young children.

Most people with fairly good digestion can start digestive enzymes at a full dose without problem, seeing only instant success. But for others, this does not work. The development of The Great Low-n-Slow Method of dosing has substantially increased the success rate with digestive enzymes. Individuals who would otherwise have quit using enzymes right away due to an intense healing crisis, have followed this program and gone on to enjoy many improvements in health and quality of life.

Enzyme dosing

Keep in mind there is not just one right way to start enzymes or dose enzymes. Many different schemes work just fine. Most people with reasonably good health do fine taking enzymes according to the recommended dosing given on the label of their chosen enzyme product from the beginning. Check the serving size or dose given on the label and use that as a guide. Then watch the reaction and adjust the dose accordingly. Since different products can have vastly different enzyme activities, you may need to take four to six capsules of one product to equal the effectiveness of one capsule of another product.

For general digestion, enzymes are dosed by the quantity and type of food, not by age or weight. Enzymes work on contact with the amount of food present. A 2-year-old tends to need as many enzymes as a 20-year-old or a 60-year-old eating the same quantity of food. That said, individual sensitivities and digestion are also a factor. You can experiment with different doses of different products for different foods. Then go with whatever dosing scheme works out best for *you*.

For maximum digestion, the goal is to give an amount of enzymes that can break down all the food eaten in the 60 to 90 minutes the food and enzymes are together in the stomach (and possibly even longer). The enzymes will continue to break down foods as the contents of the stomach move into the intestines. However, any carbohydrates, casein, or other foods not adequately broken down in the stomach and passed into the small intestine could potentially cause a food allergy or intolerance reaction in the gut. The idea is to maximize the amount of digestion in the stomach before the food enters the intestines.

To minimize adjustment effects, start with a partial dose in the very beginning and work up to a full dose.

There are very few interactions between enzymes and other supplements or medications. But if you are on a medication, particularly a time-released one, you may want to consult your doctor or pharmacist about any possible interaction for your health situation, just to be sure. Usually enzymes make any supplements or medications more effective because of enhanced absorption and gut healing.

An interesting 'side-effect' of enzyme supplements is that a person will comment that their other supplements or medication appear to start working far better after they started taking enzymes. If you are not digesting fats well, adding in fish oils may not produce the results you were hoping for. The enzyme lipase is needed to facilitate the absorption of oils. Try adding in lipase to digest fats, the fish oils can now be properly digested, absorbed, and be of use in the body.

Maintenance versus therapeutic use

Enzymes can be used for health maintenance or for therapeutic healing. Maintenance means that you want to use enzymes to help maintain your current state of health. If you have relatively healthy digestion or just mild problems which you do not want to get worse, adding a typical good quality enzyme at meals or occasionally between meals can help you maintain your current level of health. Most of the common enzyme products on the market are produced by general supplement providers who add in some type of general enzyme product as part of their supplement line. These companies usually do not specialize in enzyme formulations or enzyme therapy.

Some companies specialize in therapeutic enzymes. There are even special enzyme lines specifically for health providers, or available by prescription. A therapeutic enzyme product means the concentration of enzymes in the product as well as the particular formulation are intended to effect a positive change in health.

For those of us who have serious health problems, or pronounced gut injury, we do not want to *maintain* the current level of health. We do not want to stay where we are. We want it to *change* and get better. So we would be looking for a product designed for therapeutic healing.

Attempting to take a non-therapeutic enzyme product (that is, one designed for maintenance needs) in high enough doses so it can produce therapeutic improvements usually does not work very well. Either the blend of enzymes is not specific enough to work on the problem at hand, or the cost becomes astronomical because it takes so many more enzyme capsules of the less potent product.

Timing - Giving enzymes to break down food

Enzymes work on contact. The enzymes must be in physical contact with an appropriate target food or substance in order to work. Enzymes are usually taken at the beginning of a meal to maximize the time they can be working on the food in the stomach. Enzymes usually come in capsules you can open or swallow, or as enterically-coated tablets you cannot open. The capsules are preferable because they can either dissolve in the stomach releasing the enzymes, or you can open the capsules and mix the enzymes with any food or drink.

Some people find they get much better results when swallowing vegetable-based capsules if they take the capsule about 20 to 30 minutes before eating to allow more time for the veggie capsules to dissolve in the stomach and release the enzymes. Other people find they get the best results by opening the capsules and mixing the enzymes with the food before eating. Other people find this does not make any difference at all. You may want to experiment a little to see which method gives you the best results.

Some people find they get much better results if they take enzymes with all food and drink, especially in the beginning weeks. This may be related to helping an injured gut to heal. As the gut heals and the immune system strengthens, less enzymes may be needed over time. Also, after a few weeks or months, you may not need to be so picky about the timing, or need enzymes with all foods. Consider that the gastrointestinal system is a dynamic place. It starts repairing any damage immediately. The estimated time for gut healing is typically between three and six months for 'average' gut injury, but can be up to 12 to18 months for 'severe' cases.

On a practical note, you should be seeing some improvement in gut health by the fifth to ninth month. If you are not seeing any improvement at all by the sixth to ninth month, and there is no known reason causing constant gut injury, it would be wise to re-evaluate your gut healing program. Whether it is diet, supplements, or whatever, something needs to be changed.

Timing - Giving enzymes for a reason other than food digestion

For getting benefits with enzymes other than food digestion, you would need to research each particular area and find out the particular dosing program and enzyme mix needed for each situation. Check with your health practitioner, the manufacturer, or a health practitioner with training in enzyme therapy for appropriate dosing and blends. Both Theramedix Enzymes and Transformation Enzymes have a list of health practitioners that use enzyme therapy as part of their program.

In general, enzymes for non-food digestion uses are taken between meals. If the label on an enzyme product says to take with meals, this means it is usually designed for food digestion. If the label says to take between meals, the product is usually intended for some non-food digestion purpose.

When an enzyme product says to take between meals or on an empty stomach, it is okay to consume a little bit of food or drink with the enzymes if you need to do this to get the enzymes down. With enzymes, 'take on an empty stomach' is a general statement. It is not meant to mean the enzymes will somehow be rendered ineffective if they come into contact with even a molecule of food. It means to avoid taking the enzymes with a major meal or substantial quantity of food.

The idea of taking enzymes between meals is so the enzymes will not be slowed down working on food breakdown. The enzymes can speed on through the digestive tract, work on any health problems there, or be absorbed into the bloodstream and get on with improving health in the body. Enzymes are like little robots that work on whatever appropriate substance they come across. If they run into some food which they can work on, they will. If not, they proceed onward until they come across a substance they can work on. If the enzyme comes upon a food or substance that is not its target, it just passes the substance by doing nothing.

Reasons enzymes are used between meals include:

- Controlling harmful yeast or bacteria
- Controlling viral problems
- Healing bruises and wounds
- Cleansing blood and internal detoxification
- Treating cancer and similar chronic illnesses
- Reducing pain and inflammation, including from arthritis, fibromyalgia, or migraines

A general recommendation for colds, typical flu, routine aches, and general illness is to take a strong protease product several times a day. I usually take three to four capsules at a time (or more) every three to four hours as a general rule of thumb. This tends to significantly decrease both the duration of the illness as well as the intensity of it.

Specifics - The Great Low-n-Slow Method

Most people with typical or mildly problematic health conditions can start a good enzyme product without problem. However, those with health situations they are trying to improve or correct with a therapeutic use of enzymes may find this does not work, or causes too much discomfort in the beginning. They simply cannot seem to get out of the starting block.

The Great Low-n-Slow Method came about pretty much as a workaround to the injured gut situation. In the past, it was commonly said 'if you have an injured gut, do not take enzymes, especially the proteases.' Even now, many protease products carry a disclaimer saying to avoid enzymes or proteases if you have gastritis or other gut injury.

So, the idea that proteases might be irritating to an injured gut is not new. However, the only alternative provided was to forego digestive enzymes altogether. If you have digestive problems, you would be the one that could benefit most from digestive enzymes. Also, considering that enzymes, particularly the proteases, are so effective at healing internal tissue, this caution presented a problem.

The Great Low-n-Slow Method seems to provide the easiest adjustment for the most people in these situations of more serious gut injury. It is a strategy to help you get up and running with enzymes. It has been quite successful in minimizing any adjustment effects, and allows healing on a gentler basis. This method is strongly recommended to assist in getting started with enzymes if you have:

- Serious gut injury or digestive problems
- Bad bacteria or yeast problems
- A young child or someone with communication issues
- Precious little tolerance for discomfort of any type

The following three main steps present a general outline of how to proceed as a 'best bet' suggestion. It outlines a process for healing at a gentle rate without overwhelming the system. You can modify it as needed for your situation.

Step 1. Start with a low protease enzyme product

A basic concept is to start with a broad-spectrum enzyme product that has very low or no protease enzymes in it. The reason is that proteases tend to be workhorses in healing. Because of this, these enzymes tend to cause the most noticeable adjustment reactions. The proteases are not necessarily harmful. It is just their healing action may be too aggressive or too uncomfortable in the beginning. Starting with a product that is very low in protease allows you to get the advantages of better food digestion and initial healing, but in a more gentle manner.

Think of a time when you may have fallen and really skinned up your knee, or other similar injury. The wounded area is hurting, the skin broken, probably bleeding. Maybe there is dirt or debris in the wounded area, or the beginning of an infection. And it hurts!

What do you do? An initial reflex is to grab the wounded site and apply pressure to counter the pain. Most of us immediately rush to clean out the wound. You know this must be done. And there is no getting out of it.

We quickly find a cloth of some kind and water, start to pat the wound, cleaning it. It hurts as we do it but we are intent on doing it anyway. Why do we keep doing it if it hurts? Because we can clearly see what is going on and we do not want infection to set in. Cleaning out the wound is necessary for getting the injured tissue to heal and thus stop causing pain as quickly as possible. Not cleaning it can delay healing and even open the way for the wound to get seriously worse.

As a last step in the cleaning procedure, we get the antiseptic. Now, we *know* the antiseptic is going to sting. We also *know* it must be done. So, taking a deep breath, you close your eyes and slap the antiseptic on quickly, hoping somehow the speed of application will lessen the pain. In a few moments, it is all over. Working quickly, yet gently helps. Even after the initial cleaning is over, the wound area is still sensitive and tender for several more days. We may even apply some bandages until the wound heals over with new skin and becomes well again.

Now, consider that this may be the exact same process happening on the inside of our bodies. Wounded tissue on the inside being like wounded tissue on the outside. But we cannot see what is going on with our insides. Protease enzymes are like the wash cloth and antiseptic. They are like the cloth cleaning the wounds and the disinfectant. Beneficial, yet in the process there may be some initial irritation, pain, or discomfort when the proteases make contact with exposed, raw yet healthy tissue and nerves. This is particularly true if the gut is very damaged or inflamed.

All of this may be very alarming if you are not prepared for it. If we did not know what the antiseptic on the skinned knee was for and why it stung, we might conclude that antiseptics are bad for skinned knees. And thus the caution for people with gastritis about taking protease enzymes. The difference is that we cannot see inside ourselves to monitor what is happening. We have to interpret any progress by what we feel and know. Healing does not usually occur overnight and some patience and steady persistence may be in order.

Proteases may do other tasks besides food breakdown, which also brings the potential for more adjustment effects. Proteases can also have an impact on bad bacteria, yeast, parasites, and viruses. So, proteases can thus contribute to greater die-off reactions. These adjustment effects eventually go away after anywhere from one day to four weeks. It sometimes takes a little longer depending upon the enzyme product and the severity of your particular problem.

One way of reducing the amount of proteases you ingest is to take really tiny amounts of an enzyme product with moderate to high amounts of protease in an effort to get the proteases down to a tolerable level. However, in doing this you would also substantially decrease the total amount of all the other enzymes in the product. This may lower the quantity of other enzymes to a point where the product was much less effective. The principal behind the low protease workaround is to separate the proteases out and dose those so you have more control over any adjustment effects.

Starting with a broad-spectrum enzyme product with low or no proteases allows some gentle gut healing to occur without having to give up all the digestive action from other enzymes. By taking enough of all the other non-protease enzymes, you can slow down or stop a lot of the poorly digested foods from being a constant source of internal irritation and food intolerance reactions. You can get some great digestion of the other food types and allow gut healing to proceed at a reasonable, yet gentle rate. It also helps the body to get adjusted to improved food breakdown and nutrient absorption before the strong proteases, and more intense healing, come into play.

After some gut healing has been established, the idea is to eventually add in protease enzymes as the second step.

A 'broad-spectrum' enzyme product is one that has a variety of several different enzymes intended to help across the board for general digestion of meals containing several food groups. A broad-spectrum product usually contains enzymes for various carbohydrates, fats, proteins, and fiberous compounds. Specialized broad-spectrum products may emphasize particular foods, such as those products containing higher amounts of enzymes for dairy digestion, vegetables, or fats. If an enzyme product leads to too much discomfort initially,

... or you just do not know what to try,

... or you want a *low or no protease product* to start with, consider one of these:

- Lacto *(Enzymedica)* - particularly good if you have problems with dairy; with children; a 'best bet'
- V-Gest (*Enzymedica*) - particularly good if you have colon problems or eat lots of fruits, vegetables, or fiber foods
- Kid's Digest *(Enzymedica)* - mixes into a liquid you drink, particularly good when dealing with swallowing problems or a child under three years old

V-Gest has good activity as a broad-spectrum product, but substantially lower proteases than other broad-spectrum enzyme products. It lists around 15,000 HUT in proteases (HUT is a measure of protease activity). 15,000 sounds like is a large number. However, most enzyme products typically contain around 1 million or more protease units. 15,000 protease units is a relatively small amount. Lacto has 25,000 protease units which, again, is very low. Lacto also has additional enzymes for complete dairy digestion.

Lacto and V-gest are often tolerated where other enzyme products are not, particularly when starting enzymes. Lacto and V-gest have no fruit-derived enzymes (papain, bromelain, actinidin, ficin), fillers, or other ingredients which eliminates possible sources of problems. Starting with one bottle of either of these products is a best bet way to get off to a good start. This is especially true, if you are not sure if you react to the fruit-derived enzymes or particular added ingredients. After you complete one bottle, you can continue with this product or switch to a different broad-spectrum product containing higher levels of proteases.

Start with one-half capsule of the broad-spectrum enzyme product at one or two meals for a couple of days. Then increase to one-half capsule with all meals and bigger snacks. You can do all snacks if you want. Some people find they get significantly better results if they give enzymes with snacks, especially in the first month or two. Do this for a couple days. Then increase to one full capsule at one or two meals for a couple days with one-half capsule at other eating times. Then increase to a one full capsule at all meals and all snacks.

If at any time, you have too much die-off or are intolerably uncomfortable, stay at that enzyme level for a few days until it levels off before increasing the dose again. If you increase the enzyme dose, and find the adjustments are just too uncomfortable, decrease the dose again and stay at the reduced dose for another day or two before trying to increase it again.

There is not any one right or wrong way to do this. It will likely depend on what adjustments or healing your body is going through as well as your own personal tolerance level for how much discomfort you are willing to put up with. If you are having adjustment effects, employing measures which facilitate detoxification may be helpful: antioxidants, epsom salts, milk thistle, activated charcoal, and bottled water are options that seem to help. Please note it is just as common to have no adjustment effects or discomfort at all. So if you just feel great the entire time, that's wonderful. You are not doing anything wrong.

After you get to one full capsule of the broad-spectrum product at each meal, continue on to the second step.

Step 2. Add in a high protease enzyme product

The second step in the gentle healing process is to add in a strong protease enzyme at meals along with the broad-spectrum enzyme. A strong protease enzyme product usually contains either only proteases, or mainly proteases. There are many types of proteases, some have a more general action and some are highly specific. You may find one protease product works substantially better for you than another one. Some good protease enzymes choices are:

- GlutenEase (*Enzymedica*)
- Peptidase Complete (*Kirkman Lab*)
- Peptizyde (*HNI*)
- ViraStop (*Enzymedica*, previously called Purify)

Start at one-half capsule at one or two meals for a couple days. If all goes well, then increase to one-half capsule at all meals and any large snacks for a couple days. If this is well-tolerated, increase again to one capsule at a couple meals for a couple days with one-half capsule at other eating times. Then when that dosage is well-tolerated, increase the protease enzymes to one capsule at all meals and large snacks.

Again, it is not necessary to worry over exact capsule amounts and the exact number of days. The point is to gradually increase the proteases as they are tolerated at a comfortable level.

If at any time you have too much die-off or are intolerably uncomfortable, hold at that enzyme level for a few days and allow your body time to adjust and process out any gunk in the system. You can even reduce the dose a bit if it is too uncomfortable. Healing takes some patience and time, although enzymes are relatively efficient.

The strong proteases are much more likely to cause die-off or adjustment effects. It is very common for someone to experience no adjustments with the low protease broad-spectrum product, and get to a full capsule within a few days. When the strong protease is added, all sort of things happen. You may not be able to increase the dose of the strong protease product to a full capsule for a couple of weeks.

Strong proteases do more direct healing work, so any adjustments might be more noticeable. The advantage of this method is you can dose the proteases more or less as you need and tolerate them without giving up all the other broad-spectrum enzymes at the same time.

After you are up to one full capsule of strong protease product and one full capsule of broad-spectrum enzymes at each meal (and possibly major snacks), there are a couple options. At this point, what you decide to do can vary greatly.

First, you might want to experiment a few days with taking more of each enzyme product with meals. Try giving two to six enzymes per meal for two to four days and see if this results in more improvement. There is not an upper limit to enzymes and some people may see more benefit in higher doses. If higher doses provide additional benefits, then you can decide if you want to continue with higher doses. If you see no additional benefits, drop back to the previous dose.

Next, if you are using Lacto, V-gest, or some other low protease product as your broad-spectrum product, you might consider switching from these lower-protease products to a broad-spectrum enzyme product that contains greater amounts of proteases. This is simply for convenience and to get more proteases in at meals. Some good broad-spectrum products which are *high in proteases* are:

- Digest Gold (*Enzymedica*)
- Elite-zyme Ultra (*Thropps Nutrition*)
- Vital-zyme Forte (*Klaire Labs, original broad-spectrum product*)
- Vital-zyme Complete (*Klaire Labs, plus more specialized enzymes*)

You can also certainly continue these original products with good success. Even if you switch to a higher protease broad-spectrum enzyme product, you may want to continue giving the specific strong protease product for additional healing. At this point, you can consider continuing on to the third step.

Step 3. Add in other enzymes for special uses

The first two steps dealt with starting enzymes with meals for food digestion. The third step is optional and progresses on to starting enzymes between meals for other types of healing. This will vary considerably depending on your particular situation and need.

Additional guidelines for yeast, bacteria, and virus control

If you have, or think you might have, a yeast or *Candida* problem, adding enzymes as part of a yeast control program has proven immensely helpful for many. Yeast control usually requires a total program approach of several factors: appropriate enzymes, plus some diet changes, plus some yeast killer, plus detoxification aids, plus a good probiotic, plus stress management. For yeast, follow the first two steps for enzymes with food given previously. Then go to the section on yeast control in Chapter 11 where the guidelines for yeast control are given in three parts. The entire process may take several weeks depending on the severity of the problem.

For bacteria problems, follow the first two steps for enzymes with food, then see the section on bacteria control in Chapter 11.

For virus control, Chapter 13 gives an overview and guidelines on what to use. Chapter 14 details the results of some practical trials with enzymes for viruses, symptoms and adjustments specific to virus control, and what other people have experienced.

Additional guidelines for pain, (auto)immune conditions, arthritis, circulatory problems, fatigue, inflammation, and similar uses

Follow The Great Low-n-Slow Method presented above even if you are interested in taking enzymes for between meal use. Many people report they see better success if they also include at least a maintenance level of enzymes with meals. Many chronic problems are exasperated by poor food digestion. Often, poor digestion and nutrient intake is part of the problem even if you are not aware of any specific digestive or food problems. Even one capsule of a good quality broad-spectrum enzyme with meals can be helpful with system-wide problems.

For non-food digestion health issues, select an enzyme product designed to assist with your particular problem. For example, seaprose is a protease enzyme that is uniquely effective in clearing out excess mucus whereas nattokinase is a protease especially effective on clearing out excess fibrin and improving circulation. Bromelain is well-known for its ability to reduce inflammation. See Chapter 12, Special Enzymes for Special Needs, for further discussion on specialized enzymes.

There is overlap in these types of enzyme products. A strong protease product originally designed for food digestion may produce some benefits on system-wide problems if you take it between meals. But it might not be nearly as effective as an enzyme specializing in the target problem. Select an enzyme blend reasonably close to your goals, but do not lose sleep splitting hairs trying to figure out which exact one and only one product you should choose.

If there is more than one product which appears to meet your objectives, the best course is to get one bottle of each product you are interested in and try it. Try one bottle of one product. Then one bottle of another one. Then go with whichever product worked the best for you. Often companies provide samples if you contact them and ask. Some offer sample or trial sizes.

Try not to let price dictate your choice as much as possible. With enzymes, cheaper does not mean better. With enzymes, you need something that works on the problem at hand. A cheaper product that does not do the job is money down the drain. Enzymes are relatively inexpensive compared to the cost of other measures to maintain your health, or that assist with a chronic illness.

However, we all live in the real world. I don't know about you, but I haven't been able to get a money tree to grow in my backyard. At the end of the day, bills need to be paid with limited resources. An avenue to keep in mind is that a few companies make therapeutic lines of enzyme products. These therapeutic blends can offer higher concentrations of enzyme activities and turn out to be more cost effective in the long run.

After you are successfully at the end of Steps 1 and 2, gradually start adding in your selected enzyme product between meals. The dosage you use will depend on the product and the program you are following. A 'therapeutic dose' is generally around nine to 12 capsules of a good enzyme product taken between meals as a minimum range. This amount is in addition to any enzymes taken with food. It may sound like a lot but in reality it is not. For some conditions, such as fibromyalgia and cancer, people report taking as many as 45 to 90 capsules or more a day. There really is not an upper limit to enzymes.

Basically, with the between-meals enzyme products, the more you take the quicker you heal. It can sound like a lot, but the good news is, enzymes at these higher doses do work. And often when there are few other alternatives. Also, these higher amounts are usually for a limited amount of time to work on a specific problem. It is not like you take this high amount forever. You may need to do this for several months to help clear a problem, or get some health back. Eventually, the goal would be to get better and then switch from a high-dose therapeutic amount of enzymes to a lower-dose maintenance amount of enzymes.

When anyone in our family becomes ill, even with a cold or flu, we take three to four protease enzyme capsules every four hours. This usually speeds recovery by at least 50% and decreases the intensity of the illness by at least that much. Then, after the illness passes, the bruise heals, the pain goes away, the bacteria infection clears, or whatever, we drop back to just maintenance doses at meals.

Gradually increase the number of enzyme capsules between meals when starting. A good reference is to take one capsule three times a day between meals initially, and then increase to two capsules three times a day between meals, and then four capsules and so on until you get to the desired level.

For serious chronic illnesses, certain health professionals and doctors use special programs of enzymes as part of the treatment. Theramedix and Transformation Enzymes are two groups making therapeutic lines of enzymes and have lists of doctors who can oversee such a program.

Additional guidelines for special diets or adding in previously eliminated foods

Follow The Great Low-n-Slow Method above. After you successfully complete Step 2, continue as follows.

The general recommendation is to get adjusted to enzymes first to ensure the enzyme product itself is well-tolerated. If you want to use enzymes while continuing a special diet, you do not need to do anything else after Step 2. Good quality enzyme products generally bring another level of improvement to any special diet.

If you are interested in adding back in previously eliminated foods, select one food at a time and test it with the enzymes. Try to test a food in a 'pure' form so you can accurately tell if the food can be eaten with enzymes. For example, to test dairy, try giving whole milk because low fat milks may have hidden artificial preservatives that may cause a negative reaction. If the person is reactive to the hidden artificial additive in the low fat milk, you may mistakenly think the enzymes are not helping with the actual milk itself. Test a piece of cheese instead of cheese pizza so the bread, tomato paste, meats, and other things in the pizza are not clouding results. After a few days testing one food, you can move on to test the next food.

This gradual deliberate method of testing one food at a time helps keep results straight. If you have pizza or a casserole and all goes well, *great*! Whatever works! But if you have pizza with an enzyme and get an unfavorable reaction, do not assume it is just the cheese, or just the gluten, or just the tomato sauce. The reaction may be due to any number of ingredients that are not tolerated. You simply will not know what is the culprit. At that point, you will need to test one ingredient at a time with the enzyme to see what is actually tolerated and what is not.

Please note that even with enzymes, there may be some foods, or food chemicals, you still cannot tolerate and need to be eliminated from the diet. Artificial additives are a common problem because they are not actual nutrition from the body's point of view. Enzymes work great on real food, but artificials are not real food.

If you are not able to resume eating previously eliminated foods and you want to, continue taking enzymes for eight or more weeks to allow more time for gut healing. Then test the foods with enzymes again. It is possible a food can be put back into the diet at a later date, just not right away. Testing foods to see if they can be put back into the diet is referred to as challenging the food or challenging the diet.

Nitrates, nitrites, and sulfites can be artificially added but also occur naturally in foods. Sometimes a person has an intolerance to these chemicals which enzymes might not help because the underlying problem is not based entirely on poor digestion. If you notice you can add back many previously omitted foods except a few, try to find out if there is a common chemical in these problem foods. An example that has commonly popped up was someone could add back in most foods with enzymes except tomatoes, bananas, and oranges. It turns out that each of these foods has a higher content of amines, a compound found naturally in those foods. A person finding they can add back all foods except these should consider they may have an amine intolerance.

In this way, starting enzymes can help you further narrow down the possibilities. They can help point out to what to consider as a next step. You can learn a lot from what is 'left over' after starting enzymes.

Special Note for GFCF diets (casein-free/gluten-free): If you want to use enzymes instead of a GFCF diet, there are several enzyme products available which have been used to successfully replace a GFCF diet.

To use as a supplement or replacement for a GFCF diet, look for an enzyme product that contains an enzyme activity known as DPP IV at a minimum. DPP IV stands for dipeptidyl dipeptidase, but that is a clunky technical name that takes up more space on a product label. Although the current trend is to list DPP IV on the product label, a few enzyme products have DPP IV activity in them but do not list DPP IV activity on the label. Examples are Lacto and Digest Gold. Some probiotic products also produce DPP IV activity when tested. You can always contact the manufacturer of an enzyme product and ask if a specific activity is not listed on the label. The extent an enzyme product can replace a GFCF diet will depend on the individual sensitivity and particular product.

In addition, you may want a product(s) that also contains some carbohydrate enzymes. Gluten and casein have a carbohydrate portion that can be a source of problems in addition to the protein portion. Remember that if the villi cells are damaged, you can lose both the DPP IV activity along with the carbohydrate disaccharidase enzymes. If you have problems tolerating casein or gluten, it might be due to the protein part, the carbohydrate part, or both parts.

Most of the original enzyme products for the gluten-casein digestion problem in autism related conditions, such as Serenaid, Peptizyde, and Peptidase Complete, target the protein part of gluten (and casein). It was necessary to take another complementary enzyme product with them to work on the carbohydrate part of gluten and similar compounds.

Then, several companies began offering broad-spectrum enzyme products with large quantities of DPP IV activity added. While these all-in-one products can work for general digestion with some extra gluten control, they tend not to be able to replace a gluten-free diet completely. It could be that either the blend was not exactly right for thorough gluten digestion, or the number of capsules you would need to take for thorough gluten digestion would be four, six, or more - much more than people typically take for a meal.

A new product called GlutenEase (*Enzymedica*) goes one step further and contains enzymes targeting both the protein and carbohydrate parts of gluten. Recent experience with consumers shows this latest innovation in enzymes for gluten is usually as effective as the other products targeting only the protein portion and can similarly eliminate the need for gluten removal by most people. It also tends to be more effective for many people probably because it is also breaking down the carbohydrate portion as well. This provides a new option allowing a person to get effective gluten (and casein) breakdown in one product instead of needing two different products. This is beneficial for snacks, small amounts of gluten, or if you need very thorough gluten digestion. Combining GlutenEase with one of the broad-spectrum enzyme products is another good mix, particularly if it contains DPP IV activity.

Quick Summary of The Great Low-n-Slow Method

Step 1 – gradually start a low protease broad-spectrum enzyme product with meals and increase until you get to at least one capsule with each meal. Then go to the next step.

examples: Lacto , V-Gest, or Kid's Digest *(Enzymedica)*

Step 2 – gradually add in a strong protease enzyme product with meals until you get to one capsule with each meal.

examples: GlutenEase or ViraStop *(Enzymedica)*; AFP Peptizyde *(HNI)*; Peptidase Complete *(Kirkman)*

> **Note 1:** When you get to 1 capsule of a low protease broad-spectrum product and 1 capsule of a strong protease, you may want to switch to a broad-spectrum product that is also high in proteases. *examples:* Digest Gold *(Enzymedica)*; Elite-zyme Ultra *(Thropps Nutritionals)*; Vital-zyme Complete *(Klaire Labs)*

> **Note 2:** If you can only afford one enzyme product, instead of adding a separate protease product, you can switch from the product used in Step 1 to a broad-spectrum that is higher in proteases. This tends not to be as effective as the two product approach, but will still work if cost is an issue.

Optional Step 3 – gradually add in other enzymes for specific needs between meals.

examples: yeast-killers (Candidase, Candex, Candizyme); enzymes for autoimmune, heart, respiratory, pain, or circulatory problems (a product with seaprose, nattokinase, serratiopeptidase, bromelain, etc.)

> **Note 3:** Even if you are primarily interested in enzymes for between meal therapeutic healing and not food digestion, results tend to be better if you take at least a maintenance dose of enzymes with meals.

CHAPTER 7

Digesting Enzyme Supplements

We all have different lifestyles, situations, physical issues, and personal preferences. Fortunately, digestive enzymes come in many forms. You can mix most enzymes in any food or drink.

"Any food or drink? Will apple juice work?"

Yes, <u>any</u> food or drink.

"Applesauce?"

Yes. You can mix the enzymes in a bit of applesauce or anything else you wish, and eat just that bite first. Or mixed into the entire amount of food. Whichever you prefer.

"What about cooked apples? Or raw apple slices?"

Yes! *Any* food or drink. Basically, the rule of thumb is however you can get the enzymes down your throat is great. The exception is the food cannot be boiling hot because high heat destroys enzymes. In general, if the food or drink is cool enough to comfortably put in your mouth, it is cool enough for the enzymes.

Remember that you do not have to pick one form for all occasions. You can mix and match. You may want to use a bulk powder, chewables, or making enzyme chocolate wafers at home, but find enzyme capsules works best when you are out. Or maybe it works best the other way around. Some children have strong personal preferences on swallowing capsules, or the taste of enzymes, or what foods they will accept mixed with enzymes. Sometimes you will find one great enzyme product from one company and another key product from another company and each comes in a different form.

The important part is to remember that enzymes need to be in contact with the substance they act on. For food digestion, take enzymes just before eating. *Note:* Pancreatic enzymes sometimes say to take after eating because they want the food to buffer the enzymes. Take enzymes between meals for non-food digestion uses, such as controlling yeast, arthritis, pain, virus control, etc.

Capsules

Most digestive enzymes come in capsules which you can simply swallow. Capsules are made either of gelatin (called gel capsules) or a vegetable cellulose blend (referred to as veggie capsules). Most supplement companies have been moving toward veggie capsules over the past 10 years for all encapsulated supplements. Enzyme capsules can usually be opened to pour out the powder. If you only use part of the enzyme powder, you can simply push the two parts of the capsule back together and save the rest of the enzymes for later.

Some enzymes are specifically intended to bypass the stomach, reach the small intestine, and be absorbed into the body. These enzymes may be in capsules or tablets sealed with an enteric coating of some kind. A newer type of enteric coating consisting of all-natural cellulose plant-based materials is available on some newer enzyme products. This is a different coating than an older synthetic type of material which may cause health problems with regular use.

Bulk powder

Some enzyme products are available in bulk powder. Most provide a little plastic scoop to measure out a serving, or alternately, different amounts as you need them. Bulk powder may be helpful if you always take enzymes by mixing the enzyme powder in food or drink. *One tip here:* keep that little white drying pouch thingy that comes with the container of enzymes in the package after you open it. When enzymes are exposed to the atmosphere, the drying pouch helps keep the enzymes dry when continuously exposed to humid air with the constant opening and closing of the container. Keeping the drying pouch in the container will help maintain enzyme potency after the bottle is opened.

Chewables

Chewable enzymes have been out for many years and may be a good option if someone has a problem swallowing capsules. Chewable enzymes are popular in pet care. There are hundreds of various brands of chewables with all sorts of flavors. Here is a short-list of brands:

- Biocore Kids Chewables (*NEC*)
- BioSet Chewable Digestive Enzymes (*Enzymes, Inc*)
- HNI chewables of certain products in the line (*HNI*)
- Nutri-Essence Chewable Enzymes (*Enzymes, Inc*)
- Transformation Ripple Effect Chewable Enzymes (*Transformation*)
- WellZymes Digestive Chewables (*Enzymes, Inc*)

What tastes good varies widely by the person. Try samples of products whenever possible. Chewables tend to have more fillers than other types of enzymes. Also, you may need many more chewable tablets to equal one serving, so check the labels closely for ingredients and serving sizes. For sensory sensitive people, the texture of chewables can be a problem as much as any taste issues. As with the bulk enzyme powder, keeping the white drying pouch in the chewable enzyme container will help maintain maximum potency.

Occassionally, some people said that crushed up enzymes sprinkled on or in food can cause the mouth to feel like it is burning or tingling. This may happen with chewables or when enzymes are mixed in a drink. *IF* this happens, just wash out the mouth with a non-enzyme containing drink after chewing the chewables to ensure there is no residual enzyme in the mouth. This 'burning' is typically caused by proteases in the enzyme product starting to breakdown some of the dead layer or cells on the skin surface. Enzymes do not harm good healthy tissue, but they do remove damaged, infected, or dead cells. If proteases linger on the skin surface for a prolonged period of time, they *may* remove the dead cells exposing the healthy skin below. This can lead to very temporary irritation.

The same situation may happen if a child is taking enzymes in a drink. He may get the drink on his upper lip, like a milk mustache. If he does not wipe his mouth off, proteases may linger and he can get what looks like a rash there. Just make sure the person wipes their mouth off if they drink enzymes this way. Using a straw will also alleviate this issue. The same sort of thing can happen in the mouth if you chew on raw pineapple or papaya fruit because of the high protease content in these fruits.

Liquids

Enzymes are usually not sold as a liquid in a bottle because water 'activates' the enzyme activity. The potency would not last long in the bottle once water came into contact with the enzymes.

Dry enzyme powder, whether from a capsule or bulk powder, can be mixed into any drink as long as it is not boiling hot. High heat destroys enzymes. If you want to add enzymes to tea, for example, wait until the drink is cool enough to put in your mouth comfortably. Chewables and tablets can be crushed and mixed into drinks, but these may not mix completely due to any binders or fillers in them.

Enzymedica company introduced a new type of enzyme powder called Kid's Digest at the time of this writing. This is a new type of formuation. The enzyme powder needs to be mixed in an acidic liquid (like orange juice, lemonade, grape juice, etc). Mixing this particular product in plain water or milk alters the taste and is not recommended.

Kid's Digest contains bicarbonate and is an effervescent much like Natural Calm magnesium is a powder that effervesces in liquid. The effervescence facilitates the immediate dispersal of the enzymes in solution. In addition, the bicarbonate may help those with acid stomach, reflux, or GERD.

Kid's Digest also contains xylitol. Xylitol is a much studied natural sweetener with notable antimicrobial properties. Xylitol is increasingly popular in children's products because it helps reduce tooth decay and harmful bacterial growth.

Pancreatic enzymes

Pancreatic enzymes are derived from pig or cattle sources (also listed as ox bile). These are like our own pancreas-produced enzymes. Pancreatic enzymes are not as stable at wide ranges in pH or temperature and are destroyed by stomach acid. Thus, they are usually enterically coated to pass through to the intestines and are not active in the stomach. However, pancreatic enzymes do work and have been used quite successfully clinically for a long time.

If you cannot have any fruit-derived or fungal- derived enzymes due to serious allergies (or other reason), here are some over-the-counter products that contain pancreatic enzymes *only*:

- Solgar Pancreatic Enzymes (*Solgar*)
- Twinlabs Pancreatin (*Twinlabs*)

There are also some prescription pancreatic enzymes that require a doctor's prescription. The best known of these are Creon or Vikoase pancreatic enzymes. Insurance might cover these if a doctor writes a prescription. Three brands of pancreatic enzymes the Cystic Fibrosis Foundation has recommended are:

- Creon (*Solvay Pharmaceuticals*)
- Pancrease (*Ortho-McNeil Pharmaceuticals*)
- Ultrase (*Axcan Scandipharm, Inc.*)

There are quite a few enzyme products containing pancreatic enzymes mixed with other non-pancreatic enzymes. Because of the pancreatic portion, these enzymes are usually enterically coated to protect the pancreatic enzymes. The plant and microbial-derived enzymes in these products would not be active in the stomach because the enteric coating prevents their release in the stomach. Wobenzym brand of enzymes are well-established, highly studied examples of this group of enzymes.

Wobenzym enzymes are not promoted for food digestion. Rather this is an older line that has long been used in higher doses in the treatment of cancer, arthritis, inflammation, viral conditions, and many other system-wide chronic illnesses.

Fruit-derived enzymes

Enzymes in general can be great! However, some one may not tolerate certain fillers, added herbs, particular ingredients, or even a particular enzyme blend. The fruit-derived enzymes (bromelain, papain) are perfectly fine enzymes which are well-studied and work well for many people. But it is also known that they can be a problem for those that are phenol sensitive, salicylate sensitive, or have detoxification problems. Children with autism, ADHD, and hyperactivity problems tend to have problems with these types of enzymes. These fruit-derived enzymes, also nick-named 'the fruity enzymes,' are cross-listed as reactive with latex allergy. If you have a latex allergy, avoid these enzymes. For more on this issue, see the chapter Sulfur, Phenols, and Epsom Salts in *Enzymes for Autism/ Digestive Health* .

If you are having difficulty tolerating an enzyme product, check to see if it contains fruit-derived enzymes. If so, try a product without the fruit-derived enzymes as a first step in troubleshooting. The web site www.enzymestuff.com maintains a list of currently available enzyme products without fruit-derived enzymes. Most of the Enzymedica line does not contain fruit-derived enzymes, although a couple products do. Wellzyme enzymes avoid fruit-derived enzymes as well.

Sometimes specialized enzyme products for special uses can be used for alternate uses. Candex (*Pure Essence*) and Candizyme (*Renew Life*) in addition to Candidase (*Enzymedica*) are all designed to target yeast overgrowth, but none of these contain fruit-derived enzymes and will work for food digestion. Pancreatic enzymes would be an option as well.

If you are looking for enzyme supplements that contain *only* enzymes derived from fruit plants, bromelain and papain can be bought individually in stores. Actinidin and ficin are rarely used and hard to find individually. Bromelain is best known as an aid for reducing inflammation. Papain is also used for inflammation in addition to aiding digestion and upset stomach.

CHAPTER 8

No Pathogen Is an Island
– Biological Population Dynamics

As the days go by, progress on the yard is coming along. There is a patch towards the rear of the backyard that appears to be coming along nicely on its own. What with all the other areas needing attention, I haven't had much chance to get back there and work with it. However, from my kitchen window I can see green filling in on the exposed bare ground with the passing days. Each day there is less brown and more green coming in nice and evenly. Yessss!!! This means I can spend more time on other areas.

A few weeks later, I went over to that patch to admire the wonderful lawn coming up on its own. The patch was now covered in a deep, rich green lush growth. But, *ugh*! There is lush growth alright, lush in weeds! What I presumed was an even covering of turfgrass turned out to be an even covering of weeds.

I felt so deceived. Those sneaky weeds tricked me into leaving them alone because from a distance they appeared to resemble the grass I wanted. If the weeds growing had been radically different in height, leaf structure, color, or other visible signs, I could have easily seen they were trouble from early on and rooted them out. But these imposters, now firmly entrenched, stretched across the ground laughing at me. Stupid weeds.

I felt about 2 inches high, and that was considerably shorter than the weeds at this point. I had fallen prey to a very common technique used in nature. A pathogen or weed that closely resembles the wanted species is more likely to survive simply because it blends in better. A pest which draws a great deal of attention to itself can more easily be targeted for elimination.

Besides having a similar appearance, being 'similar' may mean the pest thrives best on the same growing conditions as the wanted species. Or the pest has a similar biology to the preferred species. This similarity means any attempt at drastically altering the environment to drive out the pest would be equally harmful to the beneficial species. This is what happens with giving a general antibiotic that kills off all bacteria: it affects the beneficial probiotics as well.

When a pest is biologically similar, it is much harder to come up with ways to drive out the pest while favoring the growth of the beneficial species. In the digestive system, a special diet or supplement designed to kill off pathogens may also harm the beneficial microbes.

Understanding the dynamics of biological populations can help when trying to establish a healthy balance of microbes in the gut and restore digestive health. It can help explain what you are seeing, and assist in designing gut healing strategies.

Appearances can be deceiving

The microbial community in the gut is a dynamic environment, just as it is in the soil. Any living organism shares its surroundings with all the other organisms around it. The different organisms compete for food, energy, moisture, space, and other resources. On a farm, weeds species compete with crops. In the gut, probiotics compete with pathogenic bacteria. In an office environment, cubicle inhabitants compete for the donuts. Competition in this sense is neither good nor bad, it is simply a way of describing the dynamics of populations.

As conditions change, populations will increase and decrease on a regular basis because of organisms emerging, growing, and dying. Even when a population is said to be steady at a desired equilibrium, this movement happens on a regular basis. The following graph shows this pattern. Notice there is a maximum and a minimum line which the population generally stays between. The dotted line represents the average population. However, even though the total number of organisms stays within the maximum and minimum range, at any particular point in time, the population fluctuates.

Natural Fluctuation Pattern of Biological Populations

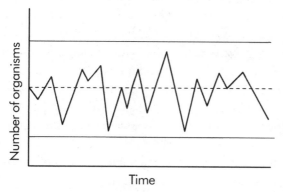

When a population is in a constant or steady state, it still falls within a range of highs and lows.

When one microbe neighborhood is abruptly disturbed through the use of any pathogen control measure, this causes a lot of shifting around among all the microbe populations. There is scrambling for new locations to populate, competition for food and fuel resources, avoidance of toxic remains, and many complicated reactions.

This shifting around can cause quite an assortment of symptoms and reactions. A person may experience a variety of reactions which change from day to day. Stools may be quite eye-opening as all sorts of gunk is being removed from the body. All of this is a typical part of eradicating pathogens. Judge how things are going over the course of several days, and not on an hour by hour basis.

Sometimes, a population can change direction slowly. Other times, the population takes a dramatic shift from its established state. The target goal in understanding population dynamics is so we can manage the populations to either stay in a healthy balance, or deliberately shift species from an unhealthy to a health-promoting level. The following example illustrates a known, natural cycle of population dynamics which may be helpful when managing microbes in our intestinal tract.

Let's say we have an area that is over-grown with a certain type of weed. We choose to use 'biological control' to manage the environment so the weed population decreases. This is similar to taking probiotics or altering the diet to deal with pathogens in the gut.

We decide to release a certain moth known to eat this particular weed while at the same time does not harm other crops or plants in the area. We release bunches of moths which promptly eat the weeds down. This dramatically lowers the weed population. The drop in weeds means the plants we want now have lots of room to use all the available resources and grow. We are thrilled with our successful plan.

However, now there are moths flying around at a certain population level. They were able to eat their fill and continue their life-cycle. They flourished and produced lots of little moths, who are also quite hungry. But now the moths' initial food supply, the weeds, is sharply depleted. While not every weed or weed seed is gone, there are not nearly enough weeds present to support the growing number of moths. The moth population starves out and dwindles down.

The low number of moths is now not sufficient to keep all the surviving weeds under control. This allows the remaining weeds to grow back again and proliferate. With insufficient moth numbers, the weeds come back in a noticeable way. At this point, we are not happy and feel our great plan has backfired.

Biological Control Dynamics

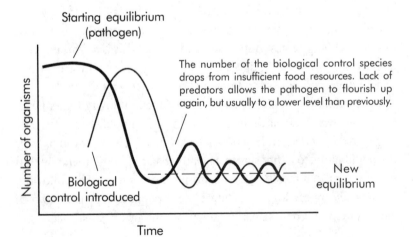

But if we are patient, the fledgling moth population once again has a food source. The moths begin to grow and reproduce as they feed on the weeds. Once more, the moths bring the weeds into check.

This cycle continues a few more times until eventually the moth and weed populations reach a new 'steady-state' or equilibrium where the moth population is in balance with a much lower weed population. The two populations go through a series of highs and lows which become less severe over time. Eventually, there are only small fluctuations in their overall population levels.

With biological control and shifting populations, ups and downs are to be expected. Often when someone does not understand this pattern, they get to the second or third cycle where the 'weeds' re-emerge, pronounce the 'treatment' a failure, and move on to something else. The person may give up in frustration before allowing enough time for the situation to reach a new steady-state.

A good example of this is when someone starts a special diet to promote good bacteria. Usually these diets call for reducing certain foods and adding in other foods in an effort to inhibit the harmful microbes and promote the beneficial microbes. These diets may include cultured foods of some type (yogurt being a prime example). Cultured foods are a whole-food source of beneficial microbes, or probiotics. Probiotic supplements are also available.

Someone following one of these diets will often report progress in their health especially in the first few months (similar to the introduction of the moths in the previous example). But later they will also report having periodic flare-ups of regression. These flare-ups are short periods where inflammation may re-appear and problems that were brought under control re-surface. While flares are known to occur with these diets, the exact cause of them is not.

What strikes me as interesting is that these flares are commonly reported to happen at distinct time-periods, such as the third, fifth, and seventh month following the beginning of the diet. The general timeframe varies depending on the specific diet and to what extent the diet is followed. It could be these flares are the resurgence of the problem microbes that caused the illness in the first place. It could be part of the up and down population cycling pattern. While the person can take different products to feel better, the flares do tend to go away on their own. This is also consistent with the ebb and flow of population dynamics. If you are not aware of this, you may be doing well on a diet or course of therapy, but get discouraged thinking the program is not working when you hit the first flare point. Then, stop the program altogether. The problem with this is that microbial ups and downs can occur with any microbial management program. So you could end up going from program to program constantly frustrated because you always hit a point where the problem microbes appear to re-bound.

A key point: altering biological populations is a *process* that may require some time and patience. If you are attempting to drive out a bad bacteria or yeast problem with probiotics, either in the form of supplements or as whole-food sources, the results may not appear to 'stick' until sometime down the road.

Another key point: it is natural to have ups and downs during the process. Having what appears to be a set-back does not necessarily mean you are doing something wrong. While it is wise to monitor what is going on, it may not be necessary to change anything, although some minor tweaking may be helpful. Also, monitor progress over longer periods of time, not on an hour by hour, or even a day by day basis. Look for overall patterns in addition to, and in balance with, individual events.

One pattern to look for when trying to correct a dysbiosis situation is to see if the more extreme highs and lows are getting less intense each time they occur. For example, you may be following a diet with the goal of reducing pathogens, and you experience periodic flare-ups where you seem to get sick again. Notice if these flare-ups get less intense each time they occur or follow any sort of pattern, such as every six weeks or every three months. Patterns and intensity levels can suggest if it is a natural course of action, or if you really need to do something different.

Probiotic populations need some time to thoroughly colonize a region in the gut. Microbial populations are not replaced all at once. Cell growth takes time. It can be days or weeks for the damaged cells to be completely replaced by healthy fully-functioning cells. Under optimal conditions, it takes a cell about five days to develop at the base of the villi and progress all the way to the tip of the villi. It takes a good three to four weeks for complete cell turnover in the digestive tract. However, with a damaged gut, conditions are not optimal. While there is healing going on from the beginning, it can take several months to really correct a bad situation.

Resisting arrest

As a farmer, you may not be able to wait several growing seasons for your biological control to reach equilibrium when you are trying to earn a living growing a crop. The bank may simply not have the same level of patience you have. In a health situation, you may not want to suffer several months waiting for your digestion to improve so you can get the nutrition you need. In the case of a growing child, it can be even harder. Other parts of the body are waiting on nutrition to come from the gut. Any waste put out by bad microbes needs to be cleared out as quickly as possible to prevent disease. Getting a bad pathogen under control quickly is a real life concern.

What if we use a type of pathogen control that kills the pathogen quickly? Instead of a 'lower-n-slower' approach we go for 'hard-n-fast?' This can work if the pathogen control measure can selectively deal a blow to only the unwanted species and spare the good guys.

In a lawn, broadleaf plants are significantly different from grass-type plants. Applying a broadleaf herbicide can effectively take out the broadleaf weeds leaving the grass safely behind. However, other weeds are grass-type weeds, such as crabgrass. A broadleaf weed control product will leave those grass weeds behind as well.

While eliminating the broadleaf weeds is interpreted as positive, there are side-effects. The resources previously used by the broadleaf weeds - nutrients, moisture, sunlight - are now available for not only the lawn grass but also the grass-type weeds. You get rid of part of the problem, but realize this may strengthen another piece of the problem. You may wake up one day shocked to find another pathogen now entrenched where the previous one was.

This can happen in the gut with certain pathogen control measures. Let's say you have a bacteria infection. You take an antibiotic. The problem bacteria are killed. But this can leave food and space for *Candida* yeast. You may not even have a *Candida* yeast problem until you take the antibiotics. It is not that it was wrong to take the antibiotic, or that the antibiotic did not work well . . . actually, it worked extremely well. The issue is there can be 'side-effect' shifts in the microbial community that leave us with less than desirable results. On a personal level, it is not that you did something wrong with your first effort, but more action is needed to bring the gut microbes into a healthy balance.

Let's say we are fed-up with all this balancing one microbe at a time, and want to start with a clean slate. We decide to strip everything out and start from scratch. An abrupt 'burndown' approach would include something like using a herbicide to kill off all the weeds and desirable plants at once, or an antibiotic that kills off all the bacteria, both good and bad. The idea is to clear out everything and start fresh, putting in only the things we want. This way only the beneficial organisms will grow and multiply, right?

This approach can be helpful in taking a huge whack at the problem, yet it is not a totally problem-free method. First, pathogens are not just flourishing on the surface, whether on the surface of the soil or on the surface in the gut. They are well-entrenched underneath as well. Sometimes very deep down. Eliminating much of the visible pathogens does not mean the environment is totally pathogen free. Know that even after an excellent start, you may very well have periodic resurgence of pathogens along the way. Pockets of resistance, so to speak. Young organisms or weed seeds will be following their life-cycle even after the initial abrupt elimination of organisms.

Another issue is that some species will change their behavior in response to their environment. If you suddenly go on a special diet in an attempt to 'starve' harmful bacteria out, some species will sense this abrupt change in their environment. In response, they start to form hard outer coverings around themselves building protective 'bunkers.' Then they enter a sort of hybernation until their enviroment becomes more favorable.

This may be a reason that a person may see initial success in controlling pathogens with a very restrictive special diet. As they try to add in new foods, the bacteria can sense their nutritional environment becoming more favorable. They emerge from their bunkers and start growing once again. The person may experience a return to their problem symptoms. This may even be a reason for flare-ups.

Casting seeds on stony ground

Even if you employ a very effective pathogen control measure, it can take a little work to get beneficial microbes established in the gut. In a post-war situation, there is still repair work and healing to be done after the fighting has ended. The environment of recently eradicated pathogens is not sitting there in optimal condition waiting to nurture new probiotics or seedlings. When the moths kill the weeds, they do not eat every molecule of the weed. The weed plant dies and you have dead weed stalks, leaves, sap, and other plant matter everywhere. This can be a big unsightly mess for a while, as well as become rather smelly as it decomposes.

In the gut, dead pathogen cells leave behind mass. Their internal cellular wastes may leach out, and even be toxic. The body needs to clear all this out. This debris can lead to the assorted unpleasant 'die-off' symptoms which accompany many pathogen control measures.

Any new probiotics or seedlings being introduced need to deal with this pathogen debris in addition to trying to get established. This may explain the difficulty seen at times when pouring probiotics into a dysbiosis situation. At times, a person laments they have been giving judicious amounts of probiotics for a year or more, either as supplements or in whole-food sources, but recent lab tests show there are no beneficial probiotics colonized in the gut. Besides being utterly frustrated at the lost expense and effort from the past year, the real need is to find out why the probiotics have not colonized and what can be done to fix the problem.

When eradicating pathogens and trying to introduce new species, the new species needs to work with the immediate environment. This immediate environment may not be healthy for the new guys. There may be chemicals and by-products in the area that are toxic to the new species. The pathogen control measure itself may have left chemical residues. The nutrients in the region, the temperature, oxygen, or pH levels in the current environment may not promote good growth. An organism may be able to survive individually, but not colonize and reproduce under the current circumstances.

Problems may exist not only from the chemical aspects of the debris, but also the physical ones. In the gut, beneficial organisms need to physically take up residence and colonize. If other organisms, dead or alive, are blocking their route or occupying their space, they will have problems adhering properly and growing. If the probiotics cannot 'stick' and grow, you can take bottles of supplements or eat tons of cultured foods, and still get a lab report showing negative adherence.

On a side note, this does not mean all those supplements, foods, or efforts were a waste. The probiotics passing through may be doing some good and give benefits. Benefits you may have seen or experienced as improved health or behavior. But the process did not progress to the point the probiotics took up residence in the gut. If you find that health is maintained only as long as you consume lots of probiotics, but drops as soon as you stop, this may explain why.

When you are trying to get a good microbial mix established in the gut, you may need to focus on different probiotic strains at different points in time. Some strains may tolerate more rugged or polluted environments. As the body is able to remove the pathogen debris and a better nutritional environment is established, you can switch to different probiotic strains. Perhaps the strains you start with are not the ones you ultimately want established. But as part of the healing process, you need a certain species first that helps clean-up the gut sufficiently for later species.

This situation can explain what happens if you try a probiotic and it is not tolerated initially. But maybe in six months or a year, you try it again and get wonderful results. Or if you initially try yogurt with live cultures or other cultured foods and have poor results. In a few months, you might try those foods again with remarkably better results.

The species you are attempting to establish has an uphill battle even without all the debris to negotiate. Consider what happens when preparing a building site. A bulldozer goes through and plows everything way under, leveling out the ground, and hauling off the big chunks of debris. If nothing else is done for weeks, nothing at all, what is the first thing to grow back? Weeds! No one needed to plant them or help them get established. They pop right up in all shapes and sizes. We do not see patches of bluegrass or manicured lawn springing up. Not even in a few small areas.

An interesting phenomenon in nature is that the unwanted species are more aggressive and robust than the wanted species (it probably has something to do with selection, survival, and the fact we tend to want more uniform populations). What this demonstrates is even with a blank slate, the hearty pathogens will attempt to make a come-back. The application of this is that an aggressive and diligent approach may be needed when putting in the beneficial organisms to help establish them as the dominant population. This applies whether trying to 'crowd out' an existing pathogen, or starting from a blank-slate.

When you are seeding a lawn, you do not put down the exact number of seeds that equal the blades of grass you want. You toss out a lot more seed knowing that only a fraction will permanently take root and survive to become part of the lawn. Even then, periodic re-seeding is needed just to maintain the lawn in good shape over time.

Healing on the go

In a lawn situation, you can strip the ground bare, and add any treatments, fertilizers, or soil tillage to prepare the area. You can plant the seeds, avoid trampling the area, and post 'stay off the grass' signs around while nurturing the new plants.

Unlike a lawn situation where you can walk away while it is being refurbished, healing a gut is something that walks with you everywhere. The process of getting the gut in good repair has to be done while you are still using it. And any problems are directly endured as you go. Another very real issue is that we cannot see directly inside ourselves to monitor the healing process to adjust our program.

While the situation is not a direct correlation, we can use basic ideas from lawn care. We cannot 'stay off the grounds' while the probiotics are trying to get established in the gut. But there are several things you can do to help ensure the 'good' bacteria can get established and keep the unwanted microbes at bay.

The previous section discussed why the beneficial species will not automatically colonize with ease just because you do not detect lots of pathogens. Patience and persistence. You will need to stick with the program, and possibly change it as you go as a normal part of the healing process.

With gut situations, you need to live with the consequences of your actions. While a more aggressive approach may drive out the pathogen faster, the die-off reaction can be so uncomfortable the person cannot tolerate it. When the treatment is with a child, the child's behavior can deteriorate to an intolerable level . . . that includes when the adults around him cannot tolerate it. Thus, it might be easier on the entire family as well as the child to go lower and slower. A 'lower-n-slower' approach tends to minimize any dramatic ups and downs. Using a lower dose of a probiotic or smaller amounts of cultured foods, and increasing the amount in a slower manner may be easier on the person in the beginning. Particularly if it is a younger child with a sensitive system.

The effects of physical stress on the immune system are another reason favoring the lower and slower approach. If the detox and die-off reactions are so severe that the immune system is overly stressed, you may not be gaining in overall health. Pathogens or other disease may gain a foothold in the body while the immune system is busy dealing with die-off reactions. Remember to keep the overall health picture in view when focusing on one aspect of your program.

You want the pathogen control program to be as aggressive as possible without overly stressing the immune system. The person needs to be able to tolerate the healing program well enough to stay with it. In practice, starting low and slow tends to work well in the very beginning. Then as healing proceeds, ramp up the program to more aggressive levels to more thoroughly correct the problem.

While starting at a low level can get one off to a great start, remaining at a low level may not be sufficient to produce a therapeutic change. That is, you will not correct the problem. The very successful Great Low-n-Slow Method, Chapter 6, outlines this process with enzymes and was developed from these principles. Guidelines for dealing with bacteria and yeast problems is given in Chapter 11.

Now, once you get a gut microbe balance in good shape, how do you keep it that way?

Mowing and mulching

A lawn is a living organism. It grows. It requires nutrients. It reproduces. It dies. I wish that once you got a lawn in perfect condition, it would just freeze that way. No maintenance. No constant fiddling with it just to keep it the same. Like artificial turf.

In lawn care, the topic of mowing and mulching frequently comes up. The general idea is to mow when there is 1/3 extra height growth. At this level of grass clippings, you can let the cuttings just fall back into the lawn where they can act as a beneficial light mulch. Appropriate mulch helps form a protective layer preventing weed growth, and can conserve moisture for the grass. The key point is the mulch is light and serves to further the growth of the lawn.

When grass is cut at no more than 1/3 of its height, the clippings are smaller. The cut pieces have much less of the woody or fibrous material present. At this size, the soil microbes in the environment can adequately breakdown the clippings, recycling the nutrients for themselves as well as for the lawn. This allows the soil microbial population to thrive in balance with the established lawn. This situation is very similar to keeping good levels of fiber in your regular diet.

Most people tend to wait until a lawn is looking a bit ragged and overgrown. Then they rev up the mower and hack away. Mowing at this grass height means you really need to catch or rake the clippings, not allowing them to fall on the grass.

When greater than 1/3 of the height is cut, the pieces are much larger and contain more fibrous plant material. Microbes in the environment have a much harder time breaking this material down and removing the chunks in a timely manner. The larger pieces laying around for a longer time can begin to kill the lawn grass creating spaces where opportunistic weeds can spring up. With enough chunkier clippings, a dense mat can form which holds in excess moisture and limits aeration. This situation promotes rot, limits the growth of the grass, and favors anaerobic disease organisms. The increasing change in environment and the promotion of other organisms alters the situation in which the initial 'good' microbes were flourishing.

In this case, you are creating a mulch, but the mulch is too dense or intense for the need. This mulch will choke out a good lawn. This situation is similar to having too much poorly digested food or fiber in the diet. Taking time to thoroughly chew your food can do wonders for overall digestion. Adding more fiber-digesting enzymes to faciliate extra fiber break down in a diet high in fiber may be helpful as well.

Going to a further extreme, if you want to prevent plant growth altogether, you can apply a thick layer of mulch, sometimes several inches thick. Using large wood chippings or bark mulches is the ultimate in hard-to-breakdown fibrous material. A heavily mulched area can provide a dense physical barrier against seedlings attempting to spring up.

Whether to mulch or not depends on what you want to accomplish. A heavy mulch surpressing lawn grass is a negative, but a heavy mulch around bushes to suppress weed growth is a positive. Also, how much mulch is present will give you very different results.

If you do some timely management practices, such as mowing at the proper time and managing the level of mulch, the lawn can stay in better shape on its own. However, life has funny ways of intruding on life. Sometimes you may not be able to get out and mow in a timely manner. Or perhaps there is a period of non-stop rainfall forcing you to mow more often than planned. Or other changes in the weather mean mowing has to be postponed until it falls during a period when you are not available. Mowing means some effort needs to be put out to keep up with the situation. However, if you do not put out this effort, even more effort will be needed later.

When the lawn is overgrown a bit, Plan B is to mow and catch the clippings so they do not over-mulch your lawn. Again, it is management appropriate to the situation. At this point, catching the clippings requires more time and effort than letting the cuttings fall into the lawn. It requires more energy, although it is also true this is some exercise many of us could use.

If the clippings are not caught and removed, the dense clippings will begin to choke out the grass. You will now need to exert even more energy to rake up the clippings and remove them. If the dense clippings are allowed to lie where they are, the situation continues to deteriorate and you will need to expend even greater effort with weed control, re-seeding, fertilization, and other measures to re-claim the lawn you once had.

Now consider how this same situation happens in our digestive tracts. With good gut health underway, if we eat wholesome foods, chew our food adequately, take a general enzyme with main meals, take a regular probiotic, and have regular elimination, this is similar to timely mowing and fertilization. It takes a little effort, but it is a basic program for maintaining good digestive health.

But if these basic steps are not pursued, the situation starts to get worse. A few episodes of constipation, a few 'junk' meals here or there, skipping the enzymes and probiotics, and similar bits of non-optimal events takes us to Plan B. Plan B means a little more effort is needed to maintain health.

If the situation is allowed to slide even further, digestive health deteriorates more and more until you are noticeably feeling bad. In the end, much more energy, effort, and even money are needed to correct the poor health situation.

The trouble is that we can see our lawn, or our lazy neighbor's, and can act. However, we cannot see inside out digestive tract. It is unwise to rely on feelings alone. By the time we 'feel' problems inside, the damage may be much worse.

Out of sight, out of mind - The making of an 'epidemic'

At times everything may seem to be just fine. A pathogen control program is going well; the microbial balance in the gut is at a healthy level. Then one day we get up and Boom! - there is a huge pathogen problem. Bacteria and yeast problems that had been vanquished have suddenly returned in force. Or a problem that seemed very minor is now abruptly out of control. When pathogen problems appear to spring up over night, or appear to surface 'all of a sudden,' this may just be the next step in a typical pathogen growth pattern.

Take the example of a lawn that is kept up reasonably well. In April, the grass is looking good. In May, it is still looking good, no weeds in sight. Come June, the view is nice, maybe a couple of solitary weeds that can easily be plucked out. In July, you gaze out and all of a sudden there are weeds all over the place. What happened?!

What happens is a typical pattern in biological population growth. A yard may harbor two weeds in the entire area. The thick, healthy lawn keeps the weeds surppressed so it is not even apparent the weeds exist. These two weeds produce a few seeds which survive. Those seeds then germinate and grow, but again, the current weed control effort is enough so you do not see those weeds. And maybe even half the weeds do not survive to reproduce. The turfgrass is still at work smothering them out.

But that still leaves half of the weeds that do survive and reproduce. Each season or cycle produces more weeds. At some point the surviving weeds become noticeable. Perhaps only a couple plants here or there appear. These can easily be plucked out if you are paying close attention. Still, they do not show much of a problem. But after that, we next see 8 plants, then 64, then 4096! Now there is a problem that needs serious attention.

The expectation that you can slowly watch a problem progressively develop over time is one based on a more liner model. However, in biology, population increases follow an exponential model. The initial stages may not be very apparent, but by the time you do see that pest, the population growth is well underway and serious.

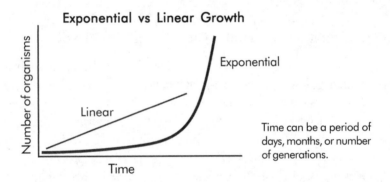

Exponential vs Linear Growth

Number of organisms

Linear

Exponential

Time can be a period of days, months, or number of generations.

Time

This is why taking proactive maintenance measures to prevent a problem before it appears is wise. Measures like a regular digestive enzyme, a regular probiotic supplement or cultured whole-foods, and making an effort to eat well on a regular basis can go along way to keeping a pathogen explosion from happening. And should you find yourself battling a pathogen outbreak, deal with it quickly to bring the gut environment back into balance.

This exponential growth works both ways. Beneficial microbes can also flourish abruptly. You may be giving a probiotic and think nothing is happening, and then one day see a sharp increase in improvements. Understanding some basic patterns in how populations work can help explain what we see when trying to achieve good digestive health. We can also use these principles to manage populations to our benefit and to achieve our goals.

Biofilms

To work with a soil, imagine you are a small microbe or root trying to gather nutrients in your immediate environment. Think of the dynamics happening on a daily basis as things pass into and out of your micro-environment. Similarly, when thinking about digestive health, imagine what a villi structure is 'seeing' in its immediate environment as it attempts to gather nutrients and ward off pathogens.

Another feature that both soils and the gut share is a very important layer called a biofilm. In the soil, the biofilm is often discussed as part of the root zone. In the gastrointestinal tract, the biofilm is often included as part of the mucosal lining.

A biofilm is a layer or coating of organic matter that harbors microbes. It is a slimy complex which develops naturally when microbes attach themselves to a substance. Some of the microorganisms produce extracellular polysaccharides and other compounds that contribute to the biofilm mix. The biofilm is a micro-environment that can provide an enhanced growing environment for the microbes such as better pH, temperature, oxygen, nutrients and other growth factors.

Biofilms may be either beneficial or harmful depending on the type of microbes involved in the biofilm. A biofilm produced by probiotics is protective in nature. A probiotic biofilm works with the intestinal environment to promote our health. A biofilm formed by harmful microbes works against the body's health.

Establishing a beneficial biofilm depends on the situation you start with. Sand or a highly sandy soil lacks the chemistry to adequately support a robust, beneficial biofilm. Sand has little organic matter so nutrients and moisture cannot be bound even as they pass by the sand particles. Sand is so loose the water slips right through it carrying nutrients away with it.

On the other hand, clay also has problems supporting a healthy biofilm, but the reason is completely different. Where sand is excessively loose, clays are too dense. The dense structure means there are very few physical spaces open to hold nutrients to support a biofilm. Roots as well as moisture have a difficult time penetrating this dense structure. Water is usually repelled away. In my yard, most of the slope as well as the ground at the base of the slope is hard clay. Water does not seep down into this soil. It either rolls right off the slope surface or puddles on top of the flat clay layer at the bottom of the hill.

Some middle ground is needed, like black loamy dirt. The black soil is balanced enough to hold an adequate amount of nutrients and water for roots to seek out as well as support a healthy biofilm. Likewise, in the gut environment, you need an appropriate biofilm to adequately mediate nutrient transfer for the villi and intestinal cells.

Earlier in this book, it was pointed out how the immediate environment of a root structure was similar to a villi structure. In both situations, the soil and the gut, you have a structure whose function is to extend out and absorb nutrition for the plant or animal. The biofilm mediates the exchange of most nutrients in both environments.

If the biofilm is too thick, nutrients will have a harder time reaching the root or villi surface. In these cases, the biofilm is seen as a barrier to nutrient uptake. Some of the special diets discuss the biofilm as being harmful because it harbors harmful bacteria. At times, a thick biofilm can protect harmful microorganisms from antibiotics, antifungals, or other pathogen control measures. However, the solution is not to try to get rid of the entire biofilm. The solution would be to replaced the harmful bacteria residing in the biofilm with beneficial probiotics and bring the biofilm back into a balance that promotes health, which is probably easier said than done.

If the biofilm is too thin, it will not be able to sustain an adequate population of beneficial microbes or protect the gut surface. A biofilm also acts as a protective layer for the root or villi. A thin biofilm may leave the root or villi surface more exposed to harmful elements.

If you read research or commercial literature, you may come across some information indicating either a biofilm is part of a health problem or it is beneficial to the health solution. Usually, the biofilm-as-a-problem is because it is either too thick or too thin under the situation discussed. The biofilm-as-beneficial view comes when the biofilm is working well and has the proper components to promote health.

With dysbiosis, the idea is to move the problem microbes and their harmful biofilm out of the gut surface and replace it with beneficial microbes. The beneficial microbes will then establish a health-promoting biofilm. This switch can take some time because the microbes are not

Impact of Benefical and Harmful Biofilms

○ Beneficial microbes (probiotics)

● Harmful microbes (pathogens)

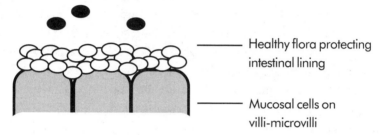

———— Healthy flora protecting
intestinal lining

———— Mucosal cells on
villi-microvilli

1. Form protective barrier inhibiting pathogens
2. By-products inhibit pathogen growth
3. Produce beneficial enzymes; aid in digestion
4. By-products stimulate immune system
5. Produce certain nutrients for human health
6. Maintain intestinal health

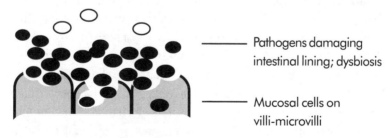

———— Pathogens damaging
intestinal lining; dysbiosis

———— Mucosal cells on
villi-microvilli

1. Form barrier inhibiting probiotics
2. By-products often toxic; damage intestinal cells
3. Invade body and infect other organs
4. Promote leaky gut; malabsorption of nutrients
5. Stress immune system
6. Detrimental to intestinal health
7. Removing microbes leaves injured cells

laying in a nice shallow row on the surface of the gut. They can be quite entrenched.

A large bush in front of our house did not survive the damage inflicted from the trenching equipment. I needed to get the 'bad' bush out and replace it with a 'good' living bush. One day I set to work digging up the 4-foot tall cone-shaped evergreen. Now, I am aware that the root system of any healthy plant below ground is generally a mirror image of whatever top growth and branching you see above ground. So that root system was going to be more cone-shaped plunging about four feet downwards. I planned on just digging out the main root ball and cut any secondary roots with the shovel instead of digging four feet down (but you know what they say about best-laid plans).

I dug down and around about 2 and a half feet, then worked on severing the roots and pulling the bush out. Nope. It was not budging because all the finer roots were so extensive holding the bush in.

I dug down and around the bush six inches more in all directions, chopping and hacking at the spindlely roots holding onto the plant. Even with my kicking and pushing on the bush, it still was not coming out. I kept digging and whacking at that frustrating shubbery until I finally got it out. In the end, the hole remaining was about four feet deep and four feet wide. At least it was large enough for the new shrub to slide right in.

Similarly in the gut, microbes may have a main mass (like the root ball). But they tend to extend out into their environment where they can. Yeast or fungal infections in particular can have long physical extending hyphae that take some effort to root out. This contributes to why yeast overgrowth is notoriously difficult to control. It can take months of steady antifungal pressure from several directions.

As the change from harmful microbes displaced by beneficial ones happens, the composition of the biofilm will change to one promoting health. The injured villi cells will be sloughed off and replaced by healthy cells. The beneficial biofilm will then be in place to help protect the gut cells. It is a back and forth dance as the healing process takes place. A steady input of probiotics, enzymes, antimicrobial factors, and other gut healing measures digs out the problem microbes and replaces them with beneficial ones.

CHAPTER 9

Probiotics - Whole-foods

Middle-school mayhem

History marks the time a certain older son of ours managed to completely disrupt the entire middle school social structure by shifting the population dynamics of his sixth grade class.

Matthew does not run with the 'popular' crowd because he would rather do other things with his free time, and he is an introvert like the rest of his family. However, just like in the movies and television shows, his class had its social structure of 'in' kids and 'out' kids with its share of the typical bully and outcast behavior.

His class used four large round tables in the lunchroom. The common routine was for all the 'popular' kids to gather at one table and gossip about or antagonize all those deemed lower than themselves at the other tables.

One day Matthew got this idea. (Now, being privy to one of Matthew's ideas can be a real treat.) He rounded up seven other classmates, all tired of being looked down on or picked on, to go along with his plan. He told everyone in their group to get in the front of the lunch-line as quickly as possible the next day so they could be first in choosing a seat at the lunch tables. Two of their group were to sit at each of the four large tables. The next day, the plan was accomplished without problem. Then, they just sat there in pairs and ate their lunch, chatting as if all was normal. That's it.

The result of this innocent sounding plan materialized when the 'popular' kids arrived in the lunchroom. As they went to take their seats, there was not one completely vacant table for them to congregate at and exclude others. So the popular kids, as they were loosely referred to, were forced to separate and mingle with those they usually avoided. Even if several of the 'in-crowd' sat at the same table, they were not about to strike up a conversation revealing all their middle school angst in front of those 'losers.' On the other hand, each 'loser' kid had a buddy for support and to talk to during lunch.

The net result? There was dead silence in the lunchroom for the entire period save some whispers, giggles, and knowing smiles by a certain pair of kids at each table. The normally rowdy lunchroom found the 'popular' kids sitting silently seething and off-balance while everyone else just sat confused or amused at all the unspoken disruption taking place.

The silence was so deafening the teachers on lunchroom duty started investigating what was going on. By mid-afternoon, most of the sixth grade teachers were involved trying to piece together what had happened. Eventually, they found the instigator of the plan.

But Mr. Creative hadn't really done anything wrong, or destructive, or . . . or . . . anything. Except in one brilliant moment he turned the entire sixth grade social structure on its head. I know this to be true because the event made its way to the principal's office who thereby contacted me to relay exactly how my son was getting along in school.

Probiotics and enzymes - Partners in digestive health

This story demonstrates how big shifts in population dynamics can result from small changes. One action can cause a ripple effect that filters through a much larger group. Population dynamics is a very intricate balance of resource allocation, compatibility, and behavior. A balance of some sort is maintained in the gut, either a balance of harmful organisms you want to disrupt, or a balance of beneficial microbes you want to maintain. A change may not even appear to be dramatic on the surface and yet it can create a huge shift in the status quo.

Enzymes are like this. By definition, enzymes are catalysts. They are proteins that can effect a large change and are not used up in the process. This is why at times you can see so many dramatic benefits from such a small amount of enzymes.

Similar dramatic changes can also come from probiotics, the beneficial bacteria that live in our guts and contribute to our health. Trillions of microorganisms live on and inside us. Some are good, some are harmful. The beneficial ones are called 'probiotic microorganisms' because they promote our health.

Probiotics work quite well with enzymes, and both are needed for good digestive health. Probiotics mainly work by improving the environment of the intestinal tract. The use of good probiotics is important in healing many chronic gastrointestinal problems. The basics of probiotics, and the evidence supporting digestive enzyme action in controlling harmful bacteria and yeast are covered in *Enzymes for Autism/Digestive Health*.

The difference in enzymes and probiotics is that enzymes are non-living proteins that do very specialized jobs repetitively, like little robots. They are eventually either eliminated from the body as part of waste products or they 'wear out' after working for a certain amount of time in the body. Probiotics, on the other hand, are living micro-organisms. They need food and fuel from their environment to survive. They reproduce and secrete by-products into their environment.

One of the very beneficial compounds probiotics manufacture are digestive enzymes. Bacteria produce and release enzymes into their immediate environment to digest substances around them to use for food. Fungi or yeasts do the same thing. While some by-products may be undesirable, the release of digestive enzymes is actually one of the main reasons probiotics are so beneficial to health.

If probiotics produce digestive enzymes, why not just take probiotics and skip enzyme supplements altogether? While probiotics can produce sufficient enzymes for their needs, the quantity of enzymes in enzyme supplements is much greater. You can get a much wider range of therapeutic amounts of enzymes from enzyme supplements. Also, supplements allow you to have much greater control over which enzymes you take and when you take them. For example, if you wanted to take more enzymes specific for fiber digestion, or viral problems, or arthritis, you would not be able to customize either the type or quantity of those specific enzymes from probiotics.

Numerous scientific studies over the last 60 years show that probiotic organisms can improve the nutritional quality of foods, produce antibiotics, anticarcinogens, and substances that break down and recycle toxins for their human host. The major benefits of adding probiotic organisms to the diet include:

- Boosting the immune system,
- Inhibiting disease causing organisms
- Improving digestion
- Synthesizing vitamins
- Removing toxins
- Preventing diarrhea from various causes
- Reducing the risk of irritable bowel syndrome and colon cancer
- Increasing nutrient absorption
- Improving resistance to allergies
- Reducing infections from harmful yeast, bacteria, and other organisms

Probiotics can be taken in whole-foods with live cultures or as probiotic supplements. Often someone will ask if they should start enzymes first or probiotic supplements. If you are already taking a probiotic, do not stop. Just add the enzymes in next. If you are not taking a probiotic or enzyme supplement, I prefer starting with enzyme supplements before probiotic supplements. Enzymes can help clear out debris and start killing off any harmful yeast or bacteria present. This provides a better environment for the probiotics when they arrive on the scene and attempt to colonize in the gut.

Think of having a lawn with lots of weeds. The enzymes act as a weed killer and the probiotics as good grass seed. Both provide benefits. But the grass will have a better chance at successfully taking root if some of the competing weeds are taken out first.

If you are considering adding probiotics in cultured whole-foods with live organisms, starting enzymes first helps you get the maximum value from the whole-foods you eat. Then after the cultured foods, consider adding probiotic supplements to boost the total amount of probiotics you consume. The reason I prioritized in this way - enzymes, whole-food probiotics, probiotic supplements - is to maximize nutritional input absorbed into the body while also maximizing debris clean-out and gut healing. However, while this is a suggested order, you may find a different order works better for you.

Probiotics in cultured whole-foods

Nutrition works best in a whole-food form. Science just doesn't understand all the intricacies of nutrient interactions yet. Taking mega-doses of one nutrient can throw another nutrient into a deficient state. If you are considering a radical change to your diet or supplement schedule, check with someone who has proper training in nutrition for your situation. You can find a registered dietician in your area at www.eatright.org (the site for the American Dieticians Association) or in the phone book.

Results from a study by Dial *et al* (1998) proved interesting on several levels. They found there were positive antibiotic properties of bovine lactoferrin on *Helicobacter pylori*, the bacteria associated with causing ulcers. They found the antibiotic benefits were greater with whole-food dairy milk than with lactoferrin supplements.

Culturing or fermenting foods is a way to get live probiotics into your diet. The fermenting process allows microbial action to partially digest the foods making them richer in available nutrients and requiring less digestive work from your body. Historically, fermentation was a method of preserving foods before refrigerators, freezers, canning, or artificial preservatives were available.

Lactic acid producing bacteria that exist on the surface of most fruits, vegetables, and other organic substances feed on the starches and sugars in food. They produce lactic acid during this feeding process. The lactic acid inhibits harmful bacteria and preserves the food. Certain yeasts can be used in the same way, such as in the making of wine and beer. In addition to lactic acid, these microorganisms produce quantities of digestive enzymes, antibiotic and anticarcinogenic substances, and other health promoting compounds. Also, the bacteria existing in food can continue to enhance digestion after you eat the cultured foods by adding beneficial bacteria into the digestive tract.

One of the most common and popular cultured foods is yogurt. Yogurt has a long history in many cultures as a foundation food. Some people do not care for the tartness of commercial yogurts, although there are many flavors available now. An alternative is to make your own yogurt, which can be cultured so it does not have this tartness. There are various recipes for making your own yogurt available online and in books. Home yogurt-makers are available for making your own yogurt, although you can certainly make it without such a gadget.

Traditionally, yogurt is made with three specific strains of probiotics: *Lactobacillus acidophilus, Lactobacillus bulgaricus,* and *Streptococcus thermophilus.* You can add in other strains if you like. Commercial yogurts may contain other strains as well.

During the culturing process, the microorganisms produce lactase enzymes and digest the lactose in dairy. They also facilitate the breakdown of dairy proteins, including casein. Research shows the lactic acid bacteria produce several aminopeptidases including the prolyl dipeptidyl dipeptidase (DPP IV). This is why someone who is lactose intolerant or has problems digesting casein can often consume yogurt without a problem. Please note commercial yogurts may not be made in the same way or have the same properties as traditionally made yogurt. Commercial yogurts may contain lactose and often have added sugar as well as other additives.

Kefir is another dairy-based fermented food. Kefir is made from *Lactobacillus acidophilus* bacteria and several different yeast organisms. The word 'kefir' comes from the Turkish word keif, meaning 'good-feeling,' 'feeling of well-being,' or 'feeling-good.' Kefir traditionally includes a dairy base, such as cow, goat, sheep, or camel's milk, but there are versions of non-dairy kefir recipes available also. Kefir is fermented using kefir grains.

To make kefir, you need some kefir grains which are commercially available or from individuals using kefir. Kefir grains are a combination of the beneficial organisms bound together in a matrix of complex sugars and casein (a milk protein). The clumps, or grains, resemble bits of cauliflower and vary in size. The kefir grains ferment the dairy they are mixed with. Afterwards, the grains are removed from the fermented dairy, and re-used in future fermentations. The principle of re-usable starter cultures is part of several whole-food probiotic foods. It is a way of manipulating bacterial growth to a favorable end.

Sourdough bread also employs a re-usable starter culture. My grandmother would keep her jar of starter in the back of the refrigerator. It had to sit and 'grow' for at least one week, and you needed to use it within three weeks time. Every two weeks she would take the starter and make several loaves of sourdough bread. And, boy, did that bread taste good! If someone wanted to make sourdough bread themselves, she would give them some of the starter from her jar.

She worked with that same jar of starter for years. Of course, the microbes in the jar had constant growth, replication, and turnover. The jar supported an ideal environment for the microbes to grow in. As with the situation with yogurt and lactose intolerance, someone who is gluten intolerant may not have any problem digesting sourdough bread because of the enzymatic pre-digestion by the microorganisms.

Sauerkraut is a familiar food, particularly popular among the brat and hotdog crowd. The traditional method of making sauerkraut is with cabbage, salt, and water. Naturally existing bacteria in and on the cabbage begin to ferment it. The salt is added to inhibit other undesirable organisms from growing. One alternative method adds yogurt or kefir grains to the cabbage mix.

There are an assortment of other vegetables and foods that can be cultured including olives, cucumbers, ginger, miso, rice, tempeh, eggplant, peppers, tomatoes, kale, beets, onion, coconut, carrots, corn, fruits, and just about anything else you care to try. *Nourishing Traditions* by Sally Fallon and Mary Enig contains recipes along with an explanation on the principles and benefits of cultured foods. *The Body Ecology* by Donna Gates also has directions for making fermented foods. The Weston A. Price organization has a great deal of information and research on eating whole-foods including cultured foods (www.westonaprice.org).

Remember that if a food is cultured, but then cooked or heated at higher temperatures, the living probiotic organisms will be killed. The resulting food will still maintain some of the benefits of the fermenting process, such as with sourdough bread, but the live organisms will no longer be reaching your digestive tract to potentially colonize there. Also, if you are using yogurt or other natural cultured food as a source of probiotics, enzymes, or other proactive healing element, this may have more of a healing 'kick' than other foods given. You may see a new round of die-off effects, or healing crises, in addition to a jump in health improvement.

What is this stuff known as milk?

Yogurt is one of the most palatable of the cultured foods, especially for children. It is a wonderful source of whole-food probiotic cultures, enzymes, minerals, lactoferrin, lysozyme, antimicrobial factors and other health enhancing compounds. Dairy consists of a variety of proteins, vitamins, minerals, other nutritious substances, and things simply called growth factors. However, there are several issues with dairy. A person may do better or worse with dairy in the diet due to any of those issues. Dairy has been alternately seen as 'liquid poison' where it is nothing but evil, and as the 'elixir of life,' the perfect food for humans as well as other animals. Either extreme wanders a bit from the truth.

Milk is a liquid that comes from the mammary glands of mammals. Other things which people sometimes call milk are usually not milk at all - such as rice milk, soy milk, potato milk, and almond milk. These are actually liquids based on plant extracts which people like to call milk because it seems to market better psychologically than something called 'plant-derived-liquid-whitish-colored-sweetened-beverage-substance.' True dairy is quite different nutritionally and constitutionally from plant extracts.

Milk is a highly studied compound because it supplies basic nutrition which baby mammals thrive on (including humans). Extensive science and research is also available from the dairy and cheese manufacturing industries.

Two enzymes in particular are associated with the digestion of dairy - lactase and DPP IV. Both enzymes originate in cells located in the mucosal lining in the intestines. If you have some type of gut injury, either of these enzymes, or both, may not be present in sufficient amounts to properly digest dairy. Supplementing these enzymes has proved quite helpful in sufficiently digesting dairy, including cultured dairy products, so they can be added back into the diet.

The milk protein casein

One category of proteins in dairy is called casein. There are a variety of different types of casein proteins in milk. Casein is also the main protein in cheese. Casein has a variety of properties, and many are quite beneficial. Calming the nervous system is one of these effects. Some people may have difficulty thoroughly digesting casein. It may be a true allergy. However, the problem is often one of insufficient protein digestion. In these cases, if the poor digestion is addressed, then the root problem is solved and casein is no longer a problem.

Enzymes targeting this casein protein is one effective method of dealing with the insufficient digestion. The enzymes break down the peptide eliminating the problem. Another possible solution is taking steps to heal an injured gut, something enzyme supplements can also facilitate in several ways.

Some people believe poorly digested casein causes the adverse problems associated with autism conditions. When dairy is taken out of the diet, some children show improvement in their 'autistic' symptoms. However, because there are so many different aspects of dairy, removing dairy does not identify what the original cause of the problems was. Missing the underlying cause has led to many of these children returning to their original problematic behaviors after several months of being dairy-free.

The theory is that the breakdown process of the casein protein gets stuck at a particular point leaving a certain peptide fragment which could act as an 'opiate.' A peptide is simply a piece broken off from a protein. Just as a piece of glass is shattered into all sorts of sizes and shapes, proteins can be broken down into many different sizes and shapes. Each fragment having unique chemistry of its own, but all referred to as 'peptides.' With further digestive action, peptides are eventually broken down into standard amino acids.

Casein is often the basis of very nutritious foods. Here are a few of the thousands of studies on casein. Meisel (1997) and Fiat and Jolles (1989) demonstrated there are an assortment of peptides derived from casein, of which only some are opiate peptides. These assorted peptides were observed to have many beneficial and healthful properties including serving as antihypertension and antimicrobial agents.

Reid and Hubbell (1994) compared the addictive property of a casein-derived peptide to morphine, and they found that although both occupy similar receptor sites, the casein peptide did not produce an addictive response whereas the morphine did.

Other detailed studies showed opioid peptides actually trigger strong development and regeneration of nervous tissue, that is, the peptides stimulate nerve growth (Sakaguchi *et al* 2001; Ilyinsky *et al* 1987). This may have something to do with the significant level of improvement some individuals with neurological problems, including autism, experience when they put dairy and whole grains back into their diets with appropriate enzymes.

Many other studies have identified antibacterial and antiviral properties in casein (Baranyi, Thomas, and Pellegrini 2003; Recio and Visser 1999; Malkoski *et al* 2001; Pellegrini *et al* 2001; Zucht *et al* 1995; Lahov and Regelson 1996). The point is if you are consuming yogurt, cheese, or some other type of dairy, and it is working to improve your health, there may be some excellent and valid reasons dairy, including the casein, is healthful. There is much evidence to support its beneficial properties.

This is consistent with the experience of many families. Whether or not one should keep casein and gluten in the diet with enzymes is up to the individual and their situation. But it is worth noting that at times these foods are very beneficial in the diet.

This leads to the question: can going dairy or casein-free make a child more susceptible to gut bacterial or viral infection? If so, then enzymes with dairy or cultured dairy may certainly be a better alternative than eliminating these foods, if possible.

The milk sugar lactose

If you take all the casein out of milk, what you have left is called whey. Whey contains the sugar lactose. If you are lactose intolerant or have some gut injury, liquid milk may cause more adverse reactions than other dairy products because it contains more lactose. Many dairy products are low in lactose or have no lactose in them, such as cheese or traditionally made yogurt.

Also, if you have bacteria or yeast issues, the lactose sugar can be used by these organisms, so you may see a 'yeast' or bacteria overgrowth reaction with liquid dairy. Common chemicals produced by these organisms are histamine and alcohols, which may produce a response very similar to the 'phenol' reactions. All of these chemicals along with by-products from yeast and bacteria overgrowth can provoke a detoxification reaction as the body tries to process them out.

If you are wondering if you have lactose intolerance as opposed to some other problem with dairy, you may want to try one of the specific high-lactose enzyme products for dairy sold in many natural food stores. Or you may want to try one of the lactose-free special milks available in stores.

Dairy, phenols, and salicylates

Some people have problems tolerating a chemical compound known as phenols. Phenols are present in all foods to some extent. Phenols are a chemical group that can be part of any of thousands of different compounds. Salicylates are one type of phenol.

A phenol structure is a
6-sided carbon ring
plus a hydroxyl (OH) side group.

OH ⬡

A salicylate structure is a
6-sided carbon ring
plus a hydroxyl (OH) side group
plus a carboxyl (COOH) side group.

OH ⬡
COOH

Certain enzymes help with the digestion and tolerance of highly phenolic foods, namely fruits and vegetables. Although the exact mechnism is not known, one reason enzymes may help with phenolic foods is they may remove a carboxyl group and allow the compound to be processed naturally and appropriately by the body. This may contribute to why enzymes appear to work much better on phenols and salicylates in real foods versus phenolic artificial ingredients.

Although dairy is ranked as extremely low in salicylates, some milk products may be high in phenols because an artificial phenolic preservative has been added to the dairy product. This added phenolic ingredient may be what causes the red ears, night waking, and other adverse reactions reported when someone sensitive to salicylates or phenols consumes dairy.

Whole milk contains natural vitamin A as a fat-soluble vitamin. The natural vitamin A and D are removed along with the fat in low-fat milks. To replace the lost nutrition, vitamin A and D are commonly added back, and the product label usually says 'with added A and D' or has vitamin A palmitate listed. However, vitamin A is not very stable so a preservative is usually added to the vitamin A to improve its stability. This preservative is usually a phenolic compound. If you have trouble tolerating phenolic compounds, you may have a problem with dairy products containing this 'hidden' preservative.

If you suspect a problem with dairy, try switching to whole milk first and see if that is tolerated better. If so, this is a clue that you may be reacting to the phenolic additive and not the dairy itself. A few brands of low-fat milks do not use the artificial preservative, but this varies by region. You need to research each brand to find out for sure. Many dairy products like cheese, yogurt, cream cheese, etc, also tend not to contain this preservative. This is one reason these other dairy products may be better tolerated than liquid milk.

Histamine and true allergies

Dairy may provoke more histamine release in the body. Someone may not have a true allergy to dairy, yet still feel uncomfortable after eating histamine-containing or histamine-provoking foods. If the person has a high level of internal histamine already, any dairy may add to it and trigger a histamine reaction. This may be the case if dairy is tolerated some of the time but not at other times. The histamine trigger may happen because of the dairy itself, or it may be a reaction to an artificial additive in the dairy product. Using Epsom salts may help reduce unpleasant histamine reactions. Reducing artificial chemicals in foods overall may reduce the total histamine load in the body. Then, regular nutritious foods cease being a problem.

If you have problems with histamine, you may also have problems with other amine compounds. Good sleep and good mood depends on proper serotonin and melatonin function. Both of these neurotransmitters are amines. Look at foods high in amines and see if you also have problems tolerating them (such as bananas, tomatoes, oranges). If so, you start to see a picture emerge where the common denominator is poor amine function in general.

A person may have a true allergy to dairy due to any of the many proteins or other factors in dairy. This may be detected as an IgE-mediated reaction, seen as a histamine type response, or something else. Reducing other histamine triggers may help, but it could be that someone is simply allergic to dairy and needs to avoid it all the time.

Proactive healing

What sets diets that include cultured whole-foods apart from being just another very restrictive diet is the proactive healing properties of the cultured foods. Food eliminations do not necessarily heal injured gut tissue. The food eliminations may slow down the damage, stop the damage, or end immediate adverse reactions, but you are still sitting there with an injured gut. The injured gut tissue may spontaneously heal on its own . . . or not. Adding in a proactive healing element allows you to kick-start and drive healing.

Proactive healing factors proven to promote tissue recovery and regrowth include probiotics, digestive enzymes, zinc, possibly essential fatty acids, and various other items. Enzymes and probiotic supplements are proactive healing elements, whether they are contained in cultured foods or in supplements. Because cultured food has so many benefical factors in it, it is understandable that yogurt would add a kick in health improvement when it is added to a restrictive diet just as adding in probiotic or enzyme supplements tend to give a big kick in health, particularly in gut health or healing a leaky gut situation. If you are nervous about adding in dairy casein, consider taking an enzyme product for casein digestion along with the yogurt. If you are concerned about the carbohydrates in cultured foods on a restrictive carbohydrate diet, consider adding in an enzyme product that is high in carbohdyrate enzymes.

What is interesting is many people reporting great success on various restrictive diets say the real healing for them did not happen until they added in the yogurt, cultured food, and/or enzymes. This includes many autism cases where dairy was originally thought to be a problem for all those with autism. There is a parallel here between the cultured-food and enzymes. Even if someone sees some improvement with their restrictive diet, the person tends to see a noticeable jump in improvement when the yogurt/cultured food or enzymes are added.

Similarly, there is also a similar 'die-off' effect when either the yogurt/cultured food or enzymes are added. Some people report, adding the yogurt/cultured food in very slowly helps reduce die-off effects, going even as low as one tablespoon per meal in the beginning. This is very similar to starting enzymes very slowly at low doses to reduce any discomfort (The Great Low-n-Slow Method).

Oftentimes, if someone hits a 'plateau' in healing on their restrictive diet, adding in either yogurt/cultured food or enzyme supplements gives them a boost in healing up to the next level. This makes complete sense given that both sources supply enzymes and are proactive healing measures. Even the special diet foods you do eat need digesting.

In real life situations, the results vary. Some people have a dairy allergy which prevents them from adding in yogurt or other cultured dairy foods. So supplements or alternate cultured foods are their only choices. For others, the yogurt or cultured foods cannot be added in immediately, but can be added after a few months of taking enzymes and probiotic supplements. In other cases, the yogurt/cultured food is only tolerated if an enzyme for dairy digestion or other appropriate enzyme is taken at the same time. After more gut healing occurs, you may be able to discontinue the enzyme supplement. Some children will not eat cultured foods, so they need supplements.

Fortunately, there are choices available to meet a wide-range of situations through cultured whole-foods and supplements, providing many more people the opportunity to improve their gastrointestinal health. This should not be seen as a competition between any special diet and supplements, but rather another example of how particular options can work together for different situations. This means more people can find workable effective solutions for their situation.

CHAPTER 10

Probiotics - Supplements

Different species of probiotic bacteria colonize in different parts of the intestines (see next page). A strain called *Lactobacillus acidophilus* resides mostly in the small intestine, and *Bifidobacterium bifidum* are found in the large intestine (colon). Probiotic products are available with only single strains and also with a combination of strains. There are mixed opinions on which types of probiotic strains are 'best' and what type of product one should take.

The truth is that it probably varies depending on the individual and their health situation. Healing the gut is a process, so even one individual may find one type of probiotic is most beneficial in the beginning of the healing process while a different mix is more helpful when further along in the gut healing program. When you eventually end up with a healthy gut, you may find a different product works best for maintenance of your gut balance.

In addition to the location of probiotic action, probiotics may be either residential or transient. Resident strains can colonize in the gut and stick around for longer periods of time. Transient microbes pass through the system without adhering and colonizing. This does not mean transient species are not beneficial. Certain transient strains have strong abilities to fight infection and may be ideal particularly in the

Location in the Gastrointestinal Tract

Probiotic activity		Enzyme activity
Numerous species including Streptococcus salivarius, Actinomyces, Bacteroides, Campylobacter, Staphylococcus	**Mouth** many microbes	Amylase in saliva; mechanical breakdown and mixing
Lactobacillus, Sarcina, Yeasts	**Stomach** few microbes; most killed by stomach acid	Proteases (pepsin); any enzymes consumed with raw foods; plant and microbial-derived enzymes active here
Lactobacillus acidophilus	**Jejunum** few microbes	Pancreatic enzymes released into small intestine: proteases (trypsin, chymotrypsin), amylases, lipases; all enzyme types active
Lactobacillus acidophilus, Enterococci	**Duodenum** few microbes	
Streptococci (viridans group), Staphylococci, Lactobacilli, Streptococcus faecalis (enterococcus), others	**Ileum** large increase in microbe numbers	Intestinal enzymes active from villi cells: certain peptidases and lipases, disaccharides (lactase, sucrase, maltase, isomaltase)
Bacillus subtilis Bifidobacterium bifidum Bifidobacterium longum Lactobacillus acidophilus Lactobacillus brevis Actinomyces, Bacteroides, Coliforms, Diphtheroids, Enterococci, Fusobacterium, Staphylococci, Spirochetes, Yeasts, Pseudomonas, others	**Colon** dramatic increase in microbes	

References: Pennsylvania State University, University of Georgia, West Virginia University beginning when there is serious intestinal damage and dysbiosis. A multi-strain probiotic product may contain both types of microbes to take advantage of the strengths of each probiotic type.

Resident strains	Transient strains
Lactobacillus acidophilus	Lactobacillus casei
Lactobacillus salivarius	Lactobacillus bulgarius
Bifidobacteria bifidum	Lactobacillus yoghurti
Bifidobacteria infantis	Lactobacillus brevis
Bifidobacteria longum	Lactobacillus kefir
Steptococcus faecalis	Lactobacillus delbrueckii
Steptococcus faecium	Lactobacillus plantarum
	Streptococcus lactis
	Streptococcus thermophillus

Some people choose a single strain of friendly flora because of the proven effectiveness of that particular probiotic strain on a particular issue. For example, Culturelle is a probiotic product containing a specific strain that is particularly helpful with colon problems. These bowel problems may range from temporary traveler's diarrhea, to a persistent *Clostridia* infection, to chronic irritable bowel syndrome. If you do not have a pronounced colon problem, you can still benefit from Culturelle. It is simply that the specific properties of this probiotic are particularly effective with colon issues.

Another example is the probiotic organism *Bacillus subtilus*. This species is particularly good at degrading organic waste. It is used to remove environmental waste or sludge by decomposing it. This probiotic type may be particularly beneficial when you have a really polluted or damaged gut, such as suffering from constipation. Or in the beginning stages of cleaning up the gut. *Bacillus subtilus* can thrive better in a less-than-ideal environment, helping to remove the toxic substances better than other probiotic organisms. After it has done some clean-up work, other probiotics can be added. The improved gut environment may improve the survival and colonization rate of other probiotics. In this situation, you may choose to use a product that contains only *Bacillus subtilus*, or you may decide to go with a product that contains *Bacillus subtilus* as a main ingredient but also includes several other beneficial probiotic strains.

Knowing that *Bacillus subtilus* helps with waste removal and Culturelle specializes in the colon, if someone had constipation or colon problems, he or she may want to use either of these two types of probiotics, or even rotate them, for this particular situation.

Rotating probiotics can mean you use one bottle of one product, and then use a bottle of a different product. Or give one type of probiotic for a few days, and then give the second product for a couple days. Another method is to take one product earlier in the day, and another product later on the same day.

Packaging and date of manufacture

Besides the specific strain, some other probiotic basics are essential. Capsules are the preferred way to take probiotics because they maintain organism integrity better. Capsules provide more protection from contamination, oxygen, and moisture. If you use probiotics in bulk, keep the little white drying sachet that comes in the probiotic package in the container to help keep down moisture levels in the package.

Probiotic products are live organisms and can lose a lot of potency after four to 10 months. The date of manufacture should be right on the bottle. Probiotics last longer when they are refrigerated, although some products do not require refrigeration. Products not requiring refrigeration are said to be 'shelf stable.' However, I have been told by some of the companies making shelf stable products that even though the product does not *require* refrigeration, they may last longer if you do keep them in the fridge. If you will be using the product rather quickly this is less of an issue than if the product is being used sporadically, or has been on the store shelf for a long period of time.

Choose a probiotic that has been extensively researched with a great deal of scientific support behind it. Fortunately, there is a substantial amount of research on many probiotic strains and more is currently underway. The research will also help you decide if one strain would be particularly beneficial for your health needs.

Probiotic strength - How much activity

Probiotic strength is measured in colony forming units (CFUs). Since probiotics are living microbes, it is the activity of the product that is important, not the weight. A dead inactive organism will have weight but it will not improve health in the gut. If a product lists only milligrams of probiotics, this could be 100% dead organisms. Or it could be 70% living and 30% dead. There is no way to tell.

Generally, high therapeutic doses of probiotics are needed when first addressing gastrointestinal problems. For therapeutic benefits, references vary widely from 250 million CFUs to more than 20 billion viable organisms per day. There is no upper limit to probiotics in general. Start at a lower amount to prevent abrupt uncomfortable die-off reactions. Then increase the amount of probiotics as it is tolerated and build-up to a level you feel is most beneficial.

For persistant *Clostridia* or *Klebsiella* infections in the colon, taking three capsules of Culturelle, 20 CFU strength, works well. Or taking Culturelle plus a *Bacillus subtilus* containing product is helpful.

In some instances, taking large amounts for a shorter period of time may be helpful to help drive out a pathogen problem. While higher doses *may* be helpful, it is not always the case that more is better. Healing a bad situation is a process. Taking smaller amounts of probiotics regularly may be much more helpful than piling on really high amounts. Just like applying lighter amounts of water or fertilizer more frequently was more helpful to seedling growth than pouring on heavy amounts.

You can experiment with different doses and probiotic strains. Then go with whatever is working best for you. You may need to try several different probiotic strains before hitting the one that gives you the best results.

If you are using a probiotic product that appears to work well, but then over time it appears to lose its effectiveness, keep in mind that healing may be underway. A shift in the microbial balance may be taking place. It could be you simply do not need as much probiotic now, or that it is time to try different strains that are more effective in a different phase of the healing process.

Timing - When to take probiotics

When to take probiotics varies by brand. Always check the label and follow the recommendation of the manufacturer. Some probiotics say to take on an empty stomach; some say take with food so the food can buffer the organisms; some say take in the morning because of stomach acid content; and some can be taken anytime. The acid and salts in the gut may harm certain probiotics and manufacturers take this into account when designing their formulations and preparing the capsules. Some capsules are specially coated so the microorganisms will safely reach their destination. Others need to be taken at certain times for optimum performance for that product. Refer to the directions on the product to see when you should take that particular probiotic, or call the manufacturer of the probiotic about their specific product.

If the manufacturer is not specific and you are unsure what to do, take enzymes at the beginning of a meal, and the probiotic at the end of the meal or some other time between meals. With my family, I used probiotics that did not require to be taken with food and gave the probiotic at bedtime. It is okay to experiment a bit with probiotic timing. Try taking it with meals for a week and then taking it between meals. Go with whichever method works best for you.

Will enzymes interfere with probiotics or probiotic foods?

The enzymes in question are usually proteases. Probiotics consist mainly of proteins so there is a line of thinking that protease enzymes might break down the probiotics or make it harder for them to securely attach and anchor in the gut.

Most probiotics are not adversely affected by enzyme supplements at all. Remember that probiotics need to exist in the gut environment which is swimming in enzymes produced by your own body most of the time anyway. You want something that is robust enough to be able to survive in the natural enzyme-filled environment of the digestive tract. In addition, probiotics produce enzymes and release them into their immediate micro-environment. To what degree a probiotic responds to enzymes depends greatly on the probiotic strain in question and how it is manufactured. Some strains are totally unaffected by enzymes, whereas other strains are slightly affected, and very rarely, a probiotic organism is strongly affected. If an enzyme or probiotic product suggests it is not stable or robust enough to exist comfortably with, or be in contact with the other, look for another enzyme or probiotic product that is. There are many fine probiotic and enzyme products available without such limitations. In the end, a heathy gut depends on probiotics and enzymes working together well in close proximity on a regular basis.

Can enzymes be taken with probiotics or probiotic foods, such as the kefir, cultured vegetables, or yogurts? Yes, you can. Probiotics in food are already in a whole-food form. Probiotics thriving in cultured food are producing digestive enzymes anyway. The probiotics are already in contact with digestive enzymes. In fact, this is a major benefit of yogurt and other fermented foods: they supply digestive enzymes to your body! The probiotics in food are already hard at work digesting food even as you are eating it.

Some of the supplement makers say "Our probiotic supplements provide much higher counts of bacteria than a cup of yogurt" and "You would need to eat six cups of yogurt to equal what you get in one supplement capsule." Supplements can provide higher concentrations of different species and strains. However, many of the probiotics in the capsules may get wiped out while traveling through the gut and attempting to colonize. It is hard to say how many live organisms will actually make it to the proper site in the intestines to work and colonize.

The yogurt makers may say, "You do not need as high a culture count because the probiotics are already established and existing in a whole-food form" and "The whole-food environment provides needed co-factors and nutrients for the microorganisms that supplements may not contain." In the final tally, the yogurt culture may well outperform the supplement. In addition, the yogurt supplies other beneficial factors for human health that a probiotic supplement does not.

Both views have valid points. My personal view is not to force yourself into always choosing one source of probiotics instead of another. You may get best results using both cultured foods as well as a daily supplement. Supplements are intended to do what their name suggests. They are to support and complement whole-food nutrition.

You may find your personal situation helps you make the choice. Someone may not be able to tolerate a large amount of yogurt or cultured food in the beginning, whereas they do benefit from probiotic supplements. Or you may find that foods with live cultures are tolerated whereas supplements are not.

There are many, many probiotics on the market. A list of suggested probiotics is available at www.enzymestuff.com under The Probiotic Short-course. This list focuses on currently available products giving consistently good results and having consistent quality based on the experiences of many people using the products. The enzymestuff site also has a list outlining features and benefits of various probiotic strains.

Beneficial yeasts

Just as there are beneficial bacteria, there are beneficial 'probiotic' yeasts (or fungi). *Saccharomyces boulardii* is a beneficial non-pathogenic yeast, also known as *Saccharomyces cerevisiae* Hansen CBS 5296. *S. boulardii* is a variant of *S. cerevisiae*. These two closely related organisms are sometimes confused as the exact same species strain, and the names used interchangeably. Both are capable of conveying similar benefits to humans. *S. boulardii* is commonly called baker's yeast whereas *S. cerevisiae* is also known as brewer's yeast. There are some cautions with taking yeast supplements particularly in conjunction with certain antidepressant medications, so consult your health practitioner before starting yeast as a supplement.

Nutritional yeast is another available yeast product. The difference in nutritional yeast and brewer's yeast appears to be the originating source. While nutritional yeast is usually derived from *S. cerevisiae*, the microbes are grown on a sweet medium, such as cane sugar or molasses. The yeast is harvested after the fermentation process is complete, purified, and prepared as a supplement. Brewer's yeast is made from by-products of breweries or distilleries.

Just like harmful bacteria, there are pathogenic yeasts, like *Candida* overgrowth, that can cause serious disease. It is important to recognize that there are beneficial and harmful organisms in each general category. Beneficial yeast is one of the components in kefir.

The beneficial enzymes in many of the enzyme supplements are derived from fungal sources. In addition, yeasts are of prime importance in baking as a leavening agent. As the yeast grows in the dough, it gives off carbon dioxide gas. This gas causes the dough to rise. In addition, some yeasts are used directly as food for humans and animals because of their high nutritive value. The beneficial yeasts supply minerals, amino acids, and B-complex vitamins.

The health promoting benefits of *Saccharomyces boulardii* include protecting the digestive tract from various diseases and pathogens, possibly helping to prevent *Candida* from spreading. This probiotic yeast has been shown to help control *Clostridia difficile*, traveler's diarrhea, and relieve some of the problems associated with Crohn's disease. (Gusland *et al* 2000; Bleichner *et al* 1997; Golledge and Riley 1996; Izadnia, Wong, and Kocoshis 1998)

Supporting the colonization of friendly bacteria and nutrient absorption in the intestines is also attributed to *Saccharomyces boulardii*. *S. boulardii* has been found to increase secretory IgA, an important part of the intestinal immune system.

Castagliuolo *et al* (1999) identified a mechanism through which *S. boulardii* improved gut health by the secretion of certain proteases that digested various toxins in the digestive tract.

An interesting application of beneficial yeast exists in the marketing of fruits. One study looked at treating sweet cherries with a naturally occuring yeast to prevent various molds and bacteria from rotting the fruit before it had a chance to sell, a problem affecting around 35% of the fruit shipments. The research tested the 'beneficial' yeast alone and in combination with a fungicide. The yeast-treatment alone prevented some types of decay, mainly harmful molds, and most of the bacteria species. The combination of the fungicide plus the yeast-treatment reduced postharvest decay by 88 to 97%. Treating postharvest fruits with beneficial yeast has undergone further study with excellent results. (Spotts *et al* 1998).

A practical application of having a beneficial yeast as an option is that the yeast would not be adversely affected by an antibiotic. So if you are taking an antibiotic, supplementing with beneficial yeast along with beneficial probiotic bacteria may be helpful. And likewise, if you are taking an antifungal, know your beneficial yeast may be in jeopardy as well.

Prebiotics - Inulin and fructooligosaccharides (FOS or scFOS)

Prebiotics are compounds thought to help promote probiotic colonization and growth. Two of the most commonly used prebiotics are FOS and inulin. These are naturally occuring non-digestible oligosaccharides, a type of sugar, that help promote the growth and activity of friendly bacteria in the intestinal tract. These oligosaccharides are considered non-caloric compounds. These sugars cannot be broken down by our digestive enzymes and therefore, generally do not adversely affect blood sugar levels (research shows unclear results in the case of diabetes). (Alles *et al* 1996; Molis *et al* 1996)

However, certain bacteria can digest these naturally occuring sugars for food. Research has shown that both FOS and inulin enhance the growth of lactic acid bacteria, especially *Bifidobacteria*, and inhibit the growth of a variety of undesirable organisms (Gibson, Beaty, and Cummings 1995; Roberfroid 1993). Other benefits from prebiotics include improved butyrate production, mineral absorption, and elimination of some toxic compounds (Tomonatsu 1994; van den Heuvel *et al* 1999).

Some probiotic supplements contain the beneficial bacteria along with some FOS or inulin in one capsule to provide a selective food supply for the probiotic, helping it to get a good rapid jump on colonization and growth in the colon. Inulin and FOS are also sold as individual supplements. The intention is that adding prebiotics to a probiotic maximizes the effectiveness of whatever probiotics are present (or consumed).

Some views hold that prebiotics can promote harmful bacteria as well as beneficial organisms. While there is some research supporting this, the bulk of the research endorses the use of prebiotics to enhance health. Anecdotal reports are split in the same way. Some people feel the addition of prebiotics hampered their health, yet many others testify the prebiotics were the magic key to their improvement.

After looking at both strategies as well as relevant research, what I glean from all this is that if you have a *serious* bad bacteria problem, then it may be best to hold off on the prebiotics, particularly avoid supplementing them in large quantities. Here, the harmful bacteria are much more prevalent and could possibly use the prebiotics for their own growth. However, if your gut health is moderately poor to fair or good, then adding prebiotics may be very beneficial, promoting the probiotics and maintaining good microflora.

Here is another way to look at this. If you have a really weedy lawn, and you throw lots of seed and fertilizer on it, the weeds are so far ahead of the grass seed and so well-established, the little grass seeds cannot compete well and struggle to get established. The weeds are able to make the most use of the fertilizer.

So, you need a blast of weed-killer of some kind to really whack out the weeds. After the weeds are thinned out a bit, you can add grass seed and lots of fertilizer. Now the grass seed has a chance to compete with the weeds. The grass noticeably benefits from the fertilizer.

Considering the dose is important. There seems to be a very wide range of what is recommended for FOS and inulin. For example, a few milligrams of a prebiotic in a probiotic supplement is very different from the 5 to 15 grams or more recommended on some FOS and inulin products. In one case, it is a 'token' amount. In another, you are flooding your system with it. One scenario may work for one person, while the other one may be better for someone else.

One animal study involved two hundred and forty young male chickens and different doses of FOS. The investigation examined the effects of FOS on digestive enzyme activities and intestinal microflora and morphology. An 'average' and a 'high' level of FOS were compared against a control group. The average level of added FOS enhanced the growth of *Bifidobacterium* and *Lactobacillus*. It also inhibited *Escherichia coli* in the small intestine and excreted digested contents. The activities of amylase and total protease significantly improved compared to the control. There was also a significant increase in ileal villus height, jejunal and ileal microvillus height, and villus-height-to-crypt-depth ratios at the jejunum and ileum, and decreased crypt depth at the jejunum and ileum.

However, the high rate of FOS did not further increase any of these factors. What this says is that some FOS is helpful in significantly improving digestive enzyme activity in the gut, improving beneficial probiotic colonization, reducing levels of harmful bacteria, and improving some parameters of gut health. But above a certain level, there is no advantage in giving even more FOS, such as mega-doses. (Xu *et al* 2003)

Whether you benefit from a prebiotic or not may depend on your specific condition and how you use the prebiotic. Also, check the strains of beneficial bacteria you are considering, both in terms of the adverse organisms you want to control and the beneficial strains in your probiotic. Some strains can metabolize prebiotics much better than others. This may influence your decision and results with FOS.

My younger son had chronic bowel problems that included substantial bad bacteria overgrowth. Probiotic supplements were a main factor in restoring good gut health. He did well with an inulin product as well as fiber-digesting enzymes. We basically were starting with no good bacteria and building from scratch. It was depressing, yes, but following the treatment for encopresis worked well. Since then, keeping him on probiotics regularly, both in whole-food yogurt form and in supplements, prevented the problem from returning.

The depressing sinkhole

We stood there staring intently at the 5-foot sinkhole, both deep and wide. The boys and I were trying to decide the best method of fixing this. It was disappointing, really, as this was the second year since the yard was dug up, and the sinkhole had only gotten substantially deeper over the area where the sewer line had been buried. And wider.

"Well, I guess we could get some black dirt delivered and start filling it in. What do you think?" I moaned out loud, hoping that some new idea would fall from the sky and relieve me of this upcoming chore. This depressing thought meant hauling wheelbarrows upon wheelbarrows of soil from the front driveway to the backyard, a notable distance, all uphill. It was almost too small a job for a landscaper to bother with and we couldn't afford a professional anyway. We had gone over all the options for months. There was simply no way out of this. It had to be done. I felt sick.

Younger Son stared intently at the hole and said matter-of-factly, "I think you should embrace the power of Ugg the Magic Dolphin."

"Definitely." his brother confirmed, eyes fixed on the hole.

My train of thought was completely disrupted. "What?!' I turned toward the younger brother not sure of what I heard. Maybe double-checking would straighten this out.

"Embrace the power of Ugg the Magic Dolphin," he said with a mischievous little grin.

Nope. Didn't help. It was probably some form of teenage boy-ese language I was left out of. I stood there with a blank look on my face trying to force the words into making sense.

Then, I caught on, and started to smile. That stupid, ridiculous comment was so unexpected and so . . . incredibly *stupid*! I started to feel not nearly so sick.

"Pancakes." Matthew continued, "Ugg definitely likes pancakes."

"With jelly," added the other brother.

"Let's fill the hole with pancakes."

"And jelly."

We were all laughing now. It was the perfect fix for our problem. Well, the problem of hauling loads of soil uphill was still there. But somehow the job was much easier because we were coming up with a multitude of ideas on what could be used to fill up a sinkhole, and the likely results, while we did it. And getting started meant we were that much closer to getting finished.

The hole was a huge patch of nothing. I ended up layering in loads of black dirt with a few bags of manure compost. I also mixed in any grass clippings I could find, which our neighbors were only too happy to have us haul off from their yards. The organic matter was food for the microbes to decompose and live on. With the hole being so deep, all of this new soil mix settled some over the next couple of seasons, so I added on a few more bags of soil the next year.

After that, I seeded over the top. The layering technique worked quite well. The soil turned out rich and the grass seed just about leaped out of the ground.

CHAPTER 11

Guidelines for
Bacteria and Yeast Control

Bacteria and yeast control are discussed here together because a population of one often influences the populations of the other. The other common pathogen group is viruses which is discussed in Chapters 13 and 14. This section will present a practical basic program for dealing with these pathogens.

There are some tests one can do to find out if bacteria or yeast is a problem, but these are known not to be 100% accurate (I have heard they run about 80% accurate). Where a test may be most helpful is when you are not getting good results from your bacteria or yeast control program. The test may be able to help identify which strains or types of bacteria or yeast you are dealing with. Some bacteria or yeast treatments may specialize in controlling certain species.

Bacteria

Probiotics are present in many cultured foods such as yogurt and kefir. Humans have consumed these foods for centuries. However, bad bacteria can develop and overrun our bodies causing illness and wreak havoc with out health. A bad bacteria problem appears to be much easier to get rid of than yeast overgrowth.

Factors that promote bacteria overgrowth

- Using too many antibiotics without probiotics can lead to bad bacterial overgrowth; the harmful bacteria are usually more aggressive at coming back and re-establishing themselves
- A poor diet; eating many processed foods; artificial additives
- Poor elimination of waste, chronic constipation, not enough fiber; harmful bacteria are more successful in a polluted environment; anaerobic environments (no oxygen) tends to kill off probiotics

Eating lots of processed and prepared foods can promote harmful bacteria as well as yeast overgrowth. Many of the commonly used preservatives functionally act as antibiotics killing off both beneficial and harmful bacteria to preserve the food. However, when you ingest these preservatives, they do not automatically stop acting or working. They can continue to be the same effective preservatives killing off the more beneficial bacteria in your gut while passing through the intestines. Harmful bacteria can then gain a foothold during this window of opportunity. Antibiotics killing off the beneficial bacteria along with the bad also leave an opening for yeast to expand and grow. Reducing the levels of preservatives in the diet as well as regularly consuming probiotics, either as supplements or in whole-foods, can minimize this problem.

Common indicators of bad bacteria

- Aggression, moodiness, irritability, 'anger' for no apparent reason
- Really foul smelling stools or body odor (we are talking incredible *stench*); bad breath; stinky sweat
- Sleep problems but without inappropriate giggling or laughter
- Ammonia or sulfur odor
- Frequently occurs with constipation (painful stools, streaking or smearing in underwear, etc); see chronic constipation or encopresis sections, pages 236 and 272.

Bacteria are composed of proteins. If you need to treat a bad bacteria problem, you might want to add some strong proteases. Enzymes tend to work synergistically with antibiotics making the bacterial control more effective.

For reasons that are not fully understood, taking supplemental proteases assists in controlling harmful bacteria while not harming beneficial bacteria. Probiotics live in our digestive systems with our own naturally produced protease enzymes all the time. So, there are likely some checks and balances involved at the microbial level that help regulate which species are cleared out with proteases and which are not. In practical experience, people find adding protease enzymes greatly helps control bacteria as well as problem yeast, while not interfering with probiotics taken either in whole-foods or as supplements.

Enzymes for fighting bacteria

My son had a terrible chronic bacteria problem. We had great success with the following program using higher doses of enzymes, probiotics, and a 10-day course of an antibiotic. I used Source Naturals brand colloidal silver for 10 days as our antibiotic with brilliant success.

Part 1. Enzymes - Good success has been seen taking between nine to 18 capsules per day of a strong protease enzyme products between meals. Take a good broad-spectrum enzyme with meals. If you are getting more nutrition and energy from your food, there is less for the bacteria to use.

Part 2. Probiotics - It is important to take lots of probiotics so there is good bacteria ready to colonize in place of the harmful species. Culturelle works very well for colon bacteria such as *Clostridia and Klebsiella* (I gave one capsule of the 20 billion CFU strength Culturelle three times a day). *Bacillus subtilus* and *Lactobacillus acidophilus* are other good choices for initial probiotics. Whole-food sources will also help. However, to initially drive out harmful bacteria, you may need more robust quantities of probiotics through supplements in addition to the whole-food sources.

Part 3. Antibiotic - Usually some type of antibiotic is needed. Most antibiotics are used for 10 days, although you may need to take herbal products longer. Many prescription antibiotics are available through your doctor. Different antibiotics work on different types of bacteria in different ways. If one is not effective, try another one which may prove more effective for you. The many non-prescription antibiotics include: colloidal silver, olive leave extract, grapefruit seed extract, cranberry, Lauricidin (TM), garlic, and tea tree oil.

Take the enzymes and probiotics first for a few weeks, and then start the antibiotic product. Continue the enzymes and probiotics for at least another few weeks after the antibiotics. Should you need to take the antibiotic more than 10 days, follow the recommendation of your health practitioner.

Whether probiotics should be given along with the antibiotics depends on individual preference. One camp feels antibiotics wipe out all bacteria, so any probiotics will be killed off as well. The other side feels beneficial bacteria needs to be present in order to be the first on the scene to colonize the space available, and ward off yeast overgrowth. Situations are so individual that there is no one right way.

Personally, I continue with probiotics during the antibiotics, particularly if it is more than a 10-day antibiotic program. With a 10-day antibiotic program, I do not give probiotics for the first few days, but start the probiotics during the last four to five days of the antibiotic round. I feel it is important to have something beneficial getting established even if some of it will be killed off with the last bits of the antibiotic. This is based more on observations of attempting to get grass seed growing while killing off weeds, and my personal comfort level. It seems logical and has worked for me in the past.

Yeast - *Candida* overgrowth

Chronic yeast overgrowth is a complex issue because of the various factors involved and the many ways it affects health. Most people report that an effective treatment involves addressing and correcting the factors that predispose an individual to *Candida* overgrowth.

Factors that promote yeast overgrowth

- Use of any antibiotic without following up with probiotics
- Lower digestive acid secretion
- Poor diet; artificial additives, preservatives
- Some medications - can be hard on gut integrity

- Nutrient deficiencies
- Low or weakened immune system function - anything that weakens the immune system
- Weak or impaired liver function
- Chronic diseases, and other factors

Common indicators of yeast are:

- Yeast rashes somewhere else in the body: thrush on the tongue, athlete's food, vaginal irritation in females, jock itch in males
- Intense carbohydrate cravings
- Inappropriate uncontrollable sudden giggling or laughter (yeast by-products include alcohol so you get 'drunk-like' behavior particularly after eating carbohydrates or sweets)
- Poor sleep, sleep waking at night
- Moodiness, unexplained emotional bouts
- Odd behavior or abrupt behavior change shortly after eating
- One of the criteria for diagnosing yeast is observing if the person responds to yeast treatment. If you given an antifungal and get either a positive or negative change, this may indicate yeast. If you start a yeast-targeting enzyme product and get a sudden reaction, this may also indicate yeast overgrowth.

Yeast control usually requires a total program approach including:

- Appropriate enzymes, plus
- Good probiotics, plus
- Yeast killer(s), plus
- Diet changes, plus
- Detoxification aids, plus
- Stress management and lifestyle changes

Any one of these, or even any two or three of these, usually will not do the trick alone. Yeast control can take months upon months to really get under control. There are a variety of yeast control diets and different philosophies. Most generally agree that processed foods and sugar intake needs to be drastically reduced to limit the yeast's food supply.

Look into several of the diets and find something appropriate for you. If the special diet is so unwieldy that you cannot maintain it, you will not stick with it. It is important to do what you can, instead of doing nothing at all.

Enzymes for fighting yeast

Many people dealing with yeast have found that combining an antifungal with a yeast-targeting enzyme product gives a powerful synergistic effect on yeast. Yeast cells have tough outer shells made up of protein and cellulose. These shells may be several layers thick and present a barrier to the commonly used antifungal medications and over-the-counter supplements. The strategy of using the yeast-fighting enzymes is to decompose or break down the yeast coverings so the yeast dies directly. And alternately, the enzymes are thought to break down the coating so that antifungals can enter the yeast cells faster, act more quickly, and destroy the yeast cells more effectively. Enzymes with meals helps deprive the yeast of their food source. In addition, protease enzymes can help reduce die-off discomfort because they can further breakdown the waste and residue left by the dead yeast cells.

For yeast control, start with the first two steps of the The Great Low-n-Slow Method, Chapter 6. Next, follow these next three parts that make up the **additional program for yeast control.**

Part 1. Start a probiotic as a supplement or in whole-foods if you are not already taking probiotics.

After you add in the enzymes for food digestion (Steps 1 and 2 of The Great Low-n-Slow Method), if you are not taking a probiotic, consider adding one at this point. Probiotics are necessary to provide some beneficial microbes ready to fill in the vacancies left by the killed bad microbes. Probiotics, enzymes, and any yeast-killer all seem to have a synergistic effect on yeast and work quite well together. However, if you start them all at the same time, the die-off can be terribly overwhelming. This gradual approach provides steady yeast control pressure while minimizing personal discomfort. This is particularly helpful for children who do not really understand why they are feeling bad, which makes it easier on their caregivers as well!

Many probiotics can be taken at the same time as enzymes. Or you can take enzymes at the beginning of the meal and probiotics at the end of the meal, in-between meals, or at bedtime. Just try taking the enzymes and your chosen probiotics both ways and go with the approach that works out best for you.

Part 2. Pick a yeast-fighting enzyme product.

After you get the probiotic to an appropriate dose, the next thing to add in is a yeast-targeting enzyme product between meals. There are several successful ones available.

Products specifically designed for yeast control:

- Candex (*Pure Essence*)
- Candidase (*Enzymedica*)
- Candizyme (*Renew Life*)

These yeast enzyme products have very different formulations. If one does not work out for you, do try one of the other products before giving up altogether. A few enzymes products intended for diets high in fruits and vegetables have high levels of fiber-digesting enzymes in them. These may help some with yeast problems; however, overall these tend to not be quite as effective on yeast as those specifically designed for yeast control.

Tip: A fair amount of experience indicates that the best results tend to come from using Candidase in rotation with one of the other yeast-targeting enzyme products. To rotate enzymes, you can substitute one capsule of another yeast enzyme product instead of one of the Candidase capsules each day (example: instead of four capsules of Candidase, use three capsules of Candidase and one of another enzyme yeast product). Some people do a rotation by giving Candidase for a couple days and then a different yeast enzyme product the next day.

This rotation advantage could be because Candidase has higher amounts of synergistic blends of proteases and cellulases, two classes of enzymes found to be most helpful on yeast. The other products have a variety of other fiber and carbohydrate digesting enzymes that might be helping to mop-up residual compounds. Generally taking three capsules of Candidase and one capsule of one of the other yeast control products works well (or a similar ratio). Again, work up to this dose gradually to minimize any die-off discomfort.

When starting enzymes for yeast control, begin with one-fourth capsule between meals. The suggestion to start yeast-control enzymes at a lower dose is so you can monitor die-off reactions. Sometimes the enzymes can really take a whack at the yeast, causing abrupt die-off discomfort. Increase the dose of the yeast-targeting enzymes slowly until you are eventually giving yeast control enzymes two to three times a day. Mid-morning, mid-afternoon, and at bedtime seem to work well.

Part 3. Add a yeast fighting herb, medication, or other product.

After you are at a full dose with your yeast control enzymes (whatever amount you find works best in your situation), the next thing to add is some type of yeast killer. This may be one of the prescription antifungals or an over-the-counter herbal product, or whatever other yeast killer you prefer. Some products combine several types of yeast killers together. Some common yeast-targeting products are:

Herbs:
- Grapefruit seed extract
- Oil of oregano
- Olive leaf extract
- Caprylic acid
- Pau d'arco
- Garlic

Medications:
- Diflucan
- Fluconazole
- Nizoral
- Sporanox
- Lotrimin

Other products - add your own discoveries here:
- *Saccharomyces cerevisiae* - beneficial yeast
- _____
- _____
- _____

Add this yeast killer in at the same time as the yeast control enzymes between meals (unless the product specifies to take at a different time). Usually an hour before or two hours afterwards is considered 'between meals.' Bedtime is a very convenient time. This way the enzymes are not held up digesting food. They can go through the digestive tract and attack the yeast more directly. It is okay to eat a little food with these products if you need it to get the yeast-fighters down.

Experience shows this combination of yeast-killer plus yeast control enzymes to be highly synergistic and effective on yeast. If you choose to add more than one yeast-killer, start one product at a time so you can tell how it is working (or if it is not well-tolerated). There may very well be a synergistic reaction as more yeast-killing items are added. Starting each item gradually will lessen any dramatic die-off reactions. When yeast is bad, it can take up to six weeks or more to slowly get through the die-off phase. Going slower can make this adjustment period more tolerable so you can actually stick with it, especially with children.

Yeast diets, detoxification aids, and stress management are not detailed here. In summary, the steps for a yeast control program, starting each item gradually in a progressive order, are:

1. Start a broad-spectrum enzyme product with meals
   (this is Step 1 of The Great Low-n-Slow Method)
2. Add in a protease enzyme product with meals
   (this is Step 2 of The Great Low-n-Slow Method)
3. Add in probiotic supplement(s) or whole-food with live cultures
4. Add in yeast control enzyme(s) product between meals
5. Add in yeast killer medication(s) or herbal product(s)
   between meals

Other useful measures:
6. Change diet to favor yeast control
7. Use detoxification aids and manage die-off (next section)
8. Zinc and magnesium may also be helpful

The entire process may take several weeks to start depending on the severity of the problem. You can always try adding in even more enzymes to help drive out the pathogen and promote healing as well.

Suggestions to help manage die-off reactions

- Following The Great Low-n-Slow Method greatly reduces die-off discomfort
- Giving more proteases - such as GlutenEase, Peptizyde, Peptidase Complete, Repair, Vitalzym, ViraStop, Wobenzym, etc. between meals - around three to four capsules every three to four hours
- Giving vitamin C or other antioxidants - helps with general detoxification; start with around 1,000 mg of buffered C three times a day, vary the dosage depending on results
- Epsom salts baths - helps with calming and detoxification
- Lots of pure water - helps flush the gunk out
- Rest, rest, sleep, and more rest - helps immune system and supports overall health
- Activated charcoal - helps absorb toxins
- Good elimination - stools moving out regularly helps eliminate toxins. If constipation is a problem, consider adding some soluble magnesium and appropriate fiber to help things move along.

What causes die-off?

Think of a bull in a china shop. The bull is roaming around causing destruction with every move, with every turn. This is similar to yeast or bacteria flourishing in the gut causing damage just by growing there. Now, let's say we take aim at the problem with effective accuracy, and shoot the destructive beast. Bam! The beast drops dead. This is like using a very effective antibiotic or yeast killer.

Now the beast is no longer flailing around causing damage. However, our problems are not over. Just look at the damage to the china shop. Broken glass everywhere. Shelving destroyed. Shards and rubbish requiring careful cleanup. It isn't like the shop can instantly re-open with customers coming and going doing business as usual. No, any customers attempting to conduct business are still subject to being harmed. At the very least, they are dramatically slowed down. This is like a cell or section of tissue attempting to function properly immediately after an antibiotic or anti-fungal treatment. While it is a better situation than when the pests are growing, it still is not optimal.

Consider also that although we do not have a rampaging bull breaking things, there is this dead bovine carcass starting to decay in the middle of the shop. It needs to be removed or the stench and rotting will create even more problems.

This is what die-off is. Remember that yeast and bacteria cells have mass. When they are killed, the micro-organisms leave a dead 'body' behind. The cellular debris from those organisms still needs to be removed from the body. Also, when a pathogen is being killed, debris and material from inside the cell may squish out, or there might be by-products released. The body has to 'detoxify' and remove all this matter somehow.

The debris may invoke the immune system to act as well. While this is going on, the person may feel sick in the stomach, like he has a flu, headaches, chills, even throw up, or other common effects seen when the body is trying to fight off invaders and clear out matter that should not be inside us. Die-off reactions refers to these symptoms we experience as the body tries to clean out the gunk. The exact symptoms will vary by person. This very well-known effect can happen anytime pathogens are being removed. It is also known as the Herxheimer Reaction. Sometimes the effects are mild, but sometimes they can be so severe you cannot function at all. The reactions may affect your emotions, thinking skills, or physical health.

Enzymes, particularly the proteases, are like the workers who come into the china shop and remove the carcass, get the store cleaned up and ready for business again. Enzymes help to break down and remove the cellulase debris left by the dead yeast and bacteria cells. They help clear out rubbish so other workers can rebuild the store. In this way, digestive enzymes help to reduce problems associated with die-off reactions.

The initial reactions may be uncomfortable during this preliminary cleaning out period. It can be like really cleaning out a dirty room, stirring up dust, moving furniture around, with cleaning supplies all around. Right after you start, the room actually looks a bit messier, more cluttered, and dirtier than when you started. But by the time you finish, it is obviously much, much cleaner (and a healthier environment).

There is a thin, gray book titled *Enzyme Therapy* by Max Wolf from the 1950s. It is quite technical and talks about enzymes used systemically to treat cancer and other related conditions (not about food digestion). In the back are six black and white photographs. They show a rat with a very large external tumor. The tumor starts at about one-fourth the size of the entire rat - huge! The tumor was treated with digestive enzymes (the basis of Wobenzym enzymes) and the photos document what happened to the rat.

The first image is of the very large and repulsive tumor on the side of the rat. It looks like the poor thing cannot even stand because the tumor is so big. The second photo shows what happened right after the initial enzyme treatment. The second photo was far more disgusting-looking than the first. The rat looked much worse. I had to study the images for a bit because I could not believe the enzymes would make the rat worse. Weren't enzymes supposed to improve the situation? What was happening was the tumor was 'dying' and disintegrating after the application of enzymes, and all the infection and crud was oozing out of the decaying cells.

The third photo showed a significant reduction in the size of the tumor with a scab forming over the healing skin. The fourth and fifth images showed rapid reduction of the tumor as it shrank to one-fourth its original size. The sixth photo showed the tumor just about gone, with most of the rat's skin healed back. The text relayed that the rat made a complete recovery including all its fur growing back where the tumor had been.

They say a picture is worth a thousand words. Although I understood the healing process, these photos made a huge impression on me of what the body can be dealing with during serious 'cleaning out' or 'die-off.' Should this debris be coming out in stool, it could make for some very interesting, if not alarming, days if you are not prepared for this possibility.

Certain yeast-fighting enzyme products promote there is 'no die-off' when using these enzyme products. However, the majority of people I have talked to using these same products reported they definitely did experience die-off reactions. The people taking such a product fully expect to feel great from the very beginning. They end up completely shocked when they get standard die-off symptoms with these enzymes. The product claims say the enzymes can kill yeast with no die-off discomfort, but experience proves this is not so.

If you use such a product without die-off symptoms, great! But if you do experience die-off reactions, please do not think you did something wrong. This is common. The good news is that at least this is evidence these products do appear to be working on the yeast.

Take the 'no die-off symptoms' with a grain of salt, or the entire salt shaker, and a bit of marketing. A technical person at one supplement company relayed that the 'no die-off' is relative to the amount of total die-off usually seen with prescription antifungals where you may have a set dose of medication given at set times. With enzymes, you can lower the dose if you need to, and then add more enzymes later. You have more control over how fast you sustain die-off symptoms (or not) and can proceed at a rate that is more comfortable.

It is true that taking enzymes may lead to relatively fewer adverse die-off reactions that other yeast control measures. The reason is that the enzymes present in the product, especially the proteases, can facilitate clearing out the debris from killed yeast or bacteria cells. This leaves less debris to cause adverse reactions. But it would be quite misleading to say you are guaranteed not to experience any die-off reactions at all with enzymes.

With any pathogen control measure, you may see die-off symptoms if the die-off is happening faster than your body can remove the waste. You can always try adding in more proteases and see if this helps relieve any die-off discomfort. A general rule of thumb is to add two capsules of strong protease enzyme for each capsule of a good quality yeast-targeting enzyme.

Probiotics can cause die-off with bacteria and yeast problems for the same reasons enzymes do (remember that probiotics produce digestive enzymes). However, probiotics have other means of causing die-off in addition to making enzymes. The good microbes physically crowd out the bad microbes by moving into their 'space' and consuming nutrients for their own growth. This denies the bad microbes of food sources. Probiotics can also have anti-pathogen properties.

If a person 'reacts' to yogurt with live cultures yet does not have a problem with other sources of dairy, it could be the probiotics at work. In addition, yogurt contains even more pathogen fighting elements besides just the probiotics.

Enzymes, probiotics, and antibiotics or antifungals work together, often synergistically. Starting one thing at a time and gradually working up to the recommended dosages tends to lessen the impact of die-off so any symptoms are not as dramatic or uncomfortable.

While it may seem depressing to have to deal with die-off symptoms, there are various ways to manage what you do to greatly minimize any discomfort. The alternative is to live with the debilitating pathogens, which really is not a good plan. Planning out a systematic course of action while taking care to deal with die-off reactions may be the quickest way to get real relief.

CHAPTER 12

Special Enzymes for Special Needs

I like mulch. I like raking the wood chips, fluffing them into place. *Rake, rake, fluff. Rake, rake, fluff.* I like the woodsy smell, the texture, the way it falls and handles. *Rake, pat, pat, fluff.* I like that it is calm, and gentle, and doesn't go storming around the house complaining endlessly about how sick it is, giving a play by play commentary on exactly how fast the phlegm in its lungs is making its way inch by slimy inch up its throat while it hacks and coughs like a thunderstorm for weeks on end keeping everyone awake night after night. All the while ignoring any helpful suggestion I might offer. Mulch is quiet, mulch is peaceful. *Rake, rake, fluff. Rake, pat, pat, fluff.*

"Helloooooo! Kaaaaren!" a voice hails.

Ohhhh! Maybe if I make myself quite small, I can disappear behind this rake.

"There you are."

Too late.

"You know that MucoStop we have?" my husband said as he came barreling round the corner.

Well, yeah! How could I forget. I had been encouraging him to try that enzyme product for nearly a year. My husband has mild asthma. It used to be that when he got sick with a cold or flu, it would get entrenched in his lungs and turn into something like bronchitis or pneumonia. A simple cold was never a simple cold. It would become weeks on end of hacking, coughing, pain, mucus, and perhaps a trip to the emergency room. He reacts pretty violently to various seasonal plants as well. When he started taking enzymes regularly several years ago, most of this pretty much disappeared.

But every so often, he comes down with a dreadful cold, flu, or allergy thing. Like now. He traditionally takes a decongestant to dry out the excess mucus so he can breathe, yet it still takes a long time for him to get well. By this time, MucoStop was available and I'd heard good reports about it.

"So, what about it?" I asked looking up from my mulching and leaning on the rake.

"Well, I decided to give it a try."

Oh, so now it was his idea??? We had gone round and round on this point several times. He said he didn't think the enzymes would be 'powerful' enough to work. My position was why not try the enzymes because it could only help and he had already tried many other things. He was not having to give up anything else. It would only be adding in something as a trial which might help.

"Yeah. Well, there is some good research on some of the enzymes in it . . .," he continued.

Might be all that information I left lying around for so long. But why ruin a perfectly good story with the facts.

"So, how did it work out?" I asked, getting rather curious now since he *had* trekked all the way out here just to find me. And I just realized his coughing spasms had stopped for the first time in days.

"Well, I am really impressed. It's definitely working. I took one MucoStop and within about 15 minutes my congestion really cleared up. Good stuff. Let's keep some of this around," he announced. And just like that, he whipped around and went back inside.

I stared. I blinked. I remembered to breathe. Well, wonder of wonders! He had gone out of his way to let me know I was rii...riiii...*right*!!! Frankly, this told me volumes about how effective MucoStop was. At least my favorite husband feels better and now we can all get some sleep.

This is why I like mulch. *Rake, rake, pat, pat, fluff.*

Seaprose - Breathe freely

Mucus is defined as a clear sluggish secretion produced by the mucous membranes. Note the difference in spelling: *mucous* refers to the component of the body secreting these compounds, while *mucus* is the actual thick slimy substance produced. Mucous membranes line various parts of the body where the external environment is in contact with the internal body, such as the gastrointestinal tract, ears, eyes, throat, and lungs. The mucous membranes produce mucus, a slippery substance, to serve as a protective layer or lubricant coating the cells and glands of various membranes separating the outside environment from the internal one (the actual inside of our bodies).

In the respiratory passages, mucus aids in protecting the lung, nose, and throat tissues by trapping foreign particles that enter the respiratory passages during normal breathing. Mucus also helps prevent these tissues from drying out. The digestive tract is also lined with mucus. In the gut, mucus acts as a lubricant to help food pass through the digestive tract. Mucus also helps protect the epithelial cells in the intestines and prevents foreign materials or pathogens from getting into the body.

So all in all, mucus is quite beneficial to health and an important member of the body's defense system. However, at times excess mucus is produced and builds up during illness. This excess mucus can become a major problem. Excess mucus can lead to infection or inflammation as it becomes dense. As mucus becomes dense, it can clog respiration, thus impeding oxygen flow and the normal removal of unwanted bacteria and debris. Harmful bacteria may find a nice, moist home in which to grow as the thick mucus protects the pathogens from the immune system. The dense substance can begin to irritate the surrounding tissues as can unwanted by-products produced by the harmful bacteria. This is one source of sinus and bronchial infections.

The idea of clearing up excess mucus is not only to help the person feel more comfortable, but also to reduce inflammation and infection in the respiratory passages. Interestingly, shortly after MucoStop became available, a prescription medication that also reduces excess mucus appeared on the market (accompanied with high profile advertising).

It is important to note that both the enzymes and medications targeting the mucus problem work to reduce *excess* mucus. Some mucus is needed in the respiratory passages for proper function. The enzymes seem to have the ability to break down only the excess mucus without overdrying. My husband said the MucoStop enzymes did not 'overdry' like many of the commercial decongestants did (such as psuedo-ephedrine), and he did not experience any other side-effects.

Personally, I do not use psuedoephedrine-type products because the overdrying causes headaches, sinus pain, and disrupts my sleep in a major way. My husband said although the MucoStop helped to clear up the excess mucus immediately, reduce the pain in the nose area, and reduce the coughing so he could breathe easier and sleep, it did not help with his sinus headache.

The enzymes in MucoStop are very different than the ones in digestive enzyme products for food, or other enzymes used systemically in the body, for that matter. Mucostop is a unique blend of enzymes formulated to break down excess mucus and possibly reduce excess histamine. The active ingredient is an enzyme called seaprose. Studies show seaprose to be quite effective in targeting and breaking down excess mucus, as well as reducing inflammation (Banchini *et al* 1993; Bracale and Selvetella 1996).

Seaprose is a semi-alkaline protease derived from the microbe *Aspergillus melleus*. It was traditionally sold in a crystalline form, which means it was more concentrated. However, this crystalline form is being discontinued. The same enzyme is also available in a less concentrated non-crystalline form trademarked as Mucolase. Both seaprose and Mucolase are measured in milligrams because at this time there are no standardized measures for this particular enzyme activity. Mucolase activity may also be given as MSO units.

As is consistent with enzymes having specific jobs, a protease that is effective at digesting food protein may not be very effective for breaking down mucus protein. Seaprose is a unique enzyme which can break down several types of proteins, but also has a particular specialization in degrading mucus proteins. At least six separate studies at the time of this writing support the beneficial effect of seaprose on bronchial and sinus mucus problems. In addition, it can help with inflammation. (Even Further References section provides a list)

One study stated, "Eight days after the end of treatment with seaprose, there was still a significant beneficial effect on the viscoelasticity of mucus and a sort of 'post-mucolytic effect' can be postulated. The enzyme seaprose also has anti-inflammatory action, and since in chronic bronchitis there are variable degrees of inflammations, its beneficial long-lasting effect could also be ascribed to this concomitant action." (Braga *et al* 1992)

Another study looked specifically at the possibility of overdrying the layer of mucus present and found this was not a problem. Moretti *et al* (1993) reported 'Furthermore the (seaprose) product does not seem to affect mucus glycoprotein secretion or secretory-IgA production, meaning it does not hinder the production of beneficial mucus.'

Since MucoStop became available some years ago, I have heard many very positive reports on it. It is taken as-needed and effects can be felt fairly quickly. One mom said it allowed her daughter with asthma to finally be able to run and play on the playground instead of sitting on the sidelines. Her daughter took one capsule of MucoStop a day and gained this great quality of life. Another parent told me her son no longer had to be on a respiratory medication and regular antihistamines for constant congestion and sinus infections.

Another source of congestion is allergies which can be caused by chemicals, plants, fur, foods, changes in the seasons, or many other things. Antihistamines are often taken along with decongestants. Amylase is thought be helpful in reducing histamine levels and have antihistamine qualities that may assist those suffering from seasonal allergies or to the common symptoms of allergies. (Desser and Rehberger 1990; Much Anecdotal Experience)

Enzymes may not have specific antihistamine properties, but they may minimize allergy reactions from appearing. By that I mean, enzymes may help support overall health and reduce the discomfort in an indirect way. Or they may help eliminate the cause that is provoking the histamine production. For example, if the by-products of bacteria or yeast are contributing to the allergies, enzyme supplements may act to control the pathogens and thus reduce the overall allergic reaction. If the immune system is working overtime to fight various pathogens, the overactive immune system might be reacting to many common environmental compounds too. Enzymes may help to reduce the total load on the immune system. In doing so, the immune system can correctly handle 'real' allergens and not overreact to anything it comes into contact with.

Enteric coatings - What the best-dressed supplements are wearing

MucoStop is an enterically-coated capsule that is not meant to be opened. This product, like a growing number of enterically-coated products, does not use the older enteric coating made with shellac and other questionable materials. This is a newer type of coating made of polysaccharide (multiple sugars) type material. Enteric coatings protect the product in the stomach but release the product in the intestines. I asked one manufacturer if this meant that seaprose and other enzymes would be destroyed by the stomach acid, or was the enteric coating just extra insurance or protection for the enzymes since these enzymes were not intended to be released and work in the stomach. The answer was that the seaprose was not destroyed in the stomach acid, and it was just for added protection so people would not open the capsules and breathe in the enzyme powder (which may act on excess mucus in the nasal passages). In addition, I was told several of the clinical studies conducted on seaprose were done without any enteric coating.

This newer enteric coating is also used on some probiotic products and brands of fish oils, all of which are not intended to be active in the stomach.

Serratiopeptidase - The silkworm's secret

A cocoon keeps a creature secure inside its protective covering. At the proper time, the conversion to a butterfly becomes complete. A silkworm's cocoon is made of a single thread about 914 meters long. About 3,000 cocoons are needed to make one pound of silk (University of Arizona 2006). But how does the little creature get out of the cocoon? Does it just rip the tightly spun wrapping to shreds through brute strength? I feel pretty safe saying we can rule out a pair of very tiny little scissors. The creature has a secret - a little enzyme secret.

Silkworms rely on a digestive enzyme known as serratiopeptidase. Serratiopeptidase is a protein-digesting enzyme derived from a bacteria that exists naturally in the intestine of the silkworm. These enzymes help the silkworm to dissolve, or digest, the cocoon surrounding it.

If you find yourself affected by regular pain or chronic illness, you may want to try the silkworm's method. Serratiopeptidase enzyme is thought to be particularly helpful with reducing inflammation and pain (such as in arthritis). Several clinical studies and many anecdotal reports support serratiopeptidase's effectiveness in pain control. It is also used for its ability to break down fibrin and excess mucus in the body (see Even Further References). Serratiopeptidase is said to have even fewer adjustments effects than other enzymes.

Serratiopeptidase enzyme is known by a variety of names and alternate spellings, including: serratiapeptidase, serrapeptidase, and serratia peptidase. Some names may refer to a company's particular serratiopeptidase product. Companies also use different processing methods. This is why some serratiopeptidase products are enterically coated while others are not. However, the basic serratiopeptidase used in products is a specific non-pathogenic enzyme derived from the organism *Serratia E15*.

Serratiopeptidase is an enzyme that has gained a great deal of attention in the past twenty years, and was of some interest even earlier. A number of products featuring serratiopeptidase have been on the market for quite a while now with a good reputation of success. Here are some common products featuring serratiopeptidase either as a single enzyme or in combination with other enzymes:

- ArthroZyme (*Sedona Labs*)
- Serrapeptase (*Enerex*)
- SerraZyme (*Serrazyme*)
- SerraPlus (*Enzymedica, serratiopeptidase alone*)
- ViraStop (*Enzymedica, serratiopeptidase blend*)
- Vitalzym (*World Nutrition*)

These enzyme products are usually taken between meals and usually at therapeutic doses of 10 to 15 capsules or more a day. Some people commonly take up to 30 to 50 capsules a day. These therapeutic programs focus on much higher doses for specific chronic illnesses such as arthritis, fibromyalgia, chronic fatigue, cancer, and viruses among others. Certain health practitioners specialize in these higher dose programs. Theramedix and Transformation Enzymes are two organizations having lists of health specialists that can incorporate enzymes into a total health care program.

A few books are available that list general suggestions for enzyme programs for specific health conditions. A recent publication is the book *Enzymes: What the Experts Know!* by Tom Bohager. It contains well-balanced suggested enzyme programs for a variety of health conditions. This book is unique in that it provides clear, general categories of enzymes and the relative needed amounts. This provides a useful, workable outline for a health practitioner or you to follow while allowing the flexibility to tailor the program to your specific needs. The suggested programs are specific enough to be useful and relevant yet general enough to be flexible and individualized.

Serratiopeptidase is an enzyme derived from a bacteria in the genus called *Serratia*. Many beneficial enzymes come from bacteria, such as all the many enzymes produced by probiotics.

Just as there are many strains of other bacteria, such as the probiotic *Lactobacillus*, there are many types of *Serratia* organisms. Most of the *Serratia* strains are non-pathogenic. However, there is one strain of the *Serratia* family, *Serratia marcesens*, thought to be potentially pathogenic in humans. The Johns Hopkins Medical Institution finds the specific organism *S. marcescens* to be the only *Serratia* species that is possibly associated with any human disease (Johns Hopkins Medical Institution Department of Pathology Newsletter 1997).

The *Serratia* organism that serratiopeptidase is derived from is not the same organism as *Serratia marcesens*. Serratiopeptidase comes from an established non-pathogenic organism known as *Serratia E15* (see Even Further References section). With any new technology, there are proposed possible concerns, but any earlier concerns based on initial speculation have since been resolved for this enzyme. Serratiopeptidase is also used as an ingredient in some medications, so it has also had to go through additional levels of research and safety testing as well.

Nattokinase - Getting to the heart of the matter

Natto is a traditional Japanese food made by adding a beneficial bacteria, *Bacillus subtilus natto*, to boiled soybeans and then fermented. The *Bacillus subtilus natto* organisms produce a specific enzyme called nattokinase. The nattokinase sold in supplements is a highly refined purified extract from this same organism.

Several health benefits have been attributed to the food natto over the years. Some may be due to the fermented whole-food soybeans themselves that is rich in vitamins, amino acids, and other nutrients. However, other health benefits may result directly from the particular enzyme nattokinase. Nattokinase has been studied as an isolated enzyme since the 1980s when Dr. Hiroyuki Sumi identified it as an enzyme that could successfully dissolve blood clots associated with heart attacks and strokes. (Sumi *et al* 1987)

Blood clots consist of blood platelets and a protein known as fibrin. After body tissue sustains injury or trauma, platelets clump together with fibrin forming a 'glue' that creates a mass in the blood with the intended function of reducing or stopping excess blood loss. The fibrin clot can further form a protective scab over a wound to facilitate healing. If blood were not able to clot like this, we could bleed to death from a simple cut.

Plasmin is the naturally occurring enzyme in our body that breaks down blood clots when they are not needed, or when they form inappropriately. When bacteria, viruses, yeasts, or other various toxins are present in the blood, these unwanted invaders can trigger an inflammatory response in the body. The inflammatory response can provoke fibrin to form unnecessarily.

Unfortunately, when there is no trauma or appropriate wound for the fibrin to work on, it circulates in the blood stream eventually settling in various parts of the body. This causes 'clutter' in the body and may contribute to various illnesses. The excess fibrin can develop into harmful blood clots which may contribute to strokes, heart attacks, pulmonary embolism, and deep vein thrombosis. Excess fibrin can also reduce blood flow causing circulatory problems, and contribute to blood pressure problems.

As we age, plasmin production slows down. This means inappropriate clots will linger around longer instead of being properly broken down and cleared out. And, unfortunately again, a factor in promoting the formation of clots, fibrinogen, increases as we age. (Hager *et al* 1994; Heinrich *et al* 1994)

The enzyme nattokinase has received a lot of attention in recent decades because it uniquely works on blood clots so similarly to plasmin. Thus, it can potentially serve as a natural plasmin-replacement in function. Currently, many of the medications and treatments for problems associated with excess clotting focus on thinning the blood. These methods may improve the flow of blood around the clots, but they do not actually remove the clots which are present. Nattokinase is believed to have an advantage over blood thinners because it works naturally to enhance the body's ability to actually dissolve the excess clots without unwanted side-effects.

Nattokinase is thought to work in two ways for extended benefits not seen with common medications used for excess fibrin problems. On the preventative side, this enzyme appears to prevent excess coagulation of blood from occurring in the first place. Secondly, nattokinase is effective in dissolving existing masses of fibrin. (Suzuki *et al* 2003; Suzuki *et al* 2003)

In one study, dogs with induced blood clots were given either four capsules of nattokinase or placebo. The dogs receiving the enzyme regained normal blood circulation free of clots within five hours. The clots in the dogs receiving the placebo showed no signs of dissolving even 18 hours later. (Sumi *et al* 1990)

Both the food natto as well as the enzyme nattokinase are well studied in assisting to normalize blood pressure and clotting issues. Future research will no doubt reveal more about these important contributors to health care.

Caution on nattokinase, blood thinners, and vitamin K

There is a special situation regarding the interaction of certain blood thinning medications and vitamin K. Vitamin K is a fat soluble vitamin discovered by a Danish scientist. The name for vitamin K comes from the Danish word 'koagulering' meaning 'clotting,' or alternatively, from the German word 'koagulation.' One of the functions of vitamin K is as an essential precursor for a protein called prothrombin needed for proper blood clot formation. (Brody 1999)

A 'blood thinner' from a pharmaceutical view is something that works as an anticoagulant. These medications do not actually thin the blood by removing harmful material. The enzyme nattokinase does work to thin the blood by removing inappropriate and excess fibrin. Both measures attempt to achieve the same goal but the mode of action is different. This is an important distinction because nattokinase is not an anticoagulant and is therefore not necessarily contraindicated when taking blood thinners.

Warfarin is a common blood thinning medication. It also goes by the trade name Coumadin. Heparin and aspirin are other known therapeutic blood thinners. Warfarin works by interfering with prothrombin formation. Warfarin dosing must be carefully monitored through testing. Too much warfarin will make the blood too thin and could lead to excess bleeding whereas too little will mean the amount of medication is not effective in preventing blood clots.

People concerned with blood clotting need to be aware of the amount of vitamin K in their diet because vitamin K promotes blood clotting. Green leafy vegetables are the foods highest in natural vitamin K. The fermented food natto also has notable amounts of vitamin K. If you are considering something like warfarin, or are on such a medication, you do not need to switch to a low vitamin K diet. What is important is to keep the level of vitamin K consistent so as not to disrupt the balance created by your current steady level of medication. (Booth 1999)

Some nattokinase supplement products contain vitamin K. Others have made a point to have any vitamin K removed. When considering a nattokinase product, make sure to investigate if the product you are considering contains any vitamin K, especially if you are taking a blood thinning medication. It does not make much sense to take a nattokinase product to reduce blood clots when that same product may contain an ingredient that promotes clotting. A form of nattokinase that is specifically made to be free of vitamin K is noted as NSK-SD.

Look for products with the NSK-SD type of nattokinase if you want it without the vitamin K, such as:

Natto-K (*Enzymedica*)
Nattokinase NSK-SD (*Source Naturals*)

Catalase

When oxygen-using organisms metabolize oxygen through respiration, harmful hydrogen peroxide and free radicals are released. Fatty acid metabolism can generate hydrogen peroxide as can the action of white blood cells acting on harmful bacteria. The organism must have some way to clear these compounds out or it will be poisoned. Hydrogen peroxide is toxic and can form carbon dioxide bubbles in the blood if not controlled. Free radicals can cause havoc with DNA integrity and interfere with other cell reactions.

Catalase is a highly efficient enzyme that works to detoxify hydrogen peroxide and clear out free radicals. Catalase is a natural enzyme produced in the body for these purposes. It enhances the conversion of hydrogen peroxide to water and oxygen. Catalase also works to breakdown potentially harmful toxins such as alcohols, phenols, and formaldehydes. Super oxide dimutase, often noted as SOD, and glutathione peroxidase are two other enzymes with antioxidant properties similar to catalase.

When hydrogen peroxide is poured on a cut, the catalase in our tissues breaks it down as it works. The release of the oxygen causes the hydrogen peroxide to foam when applied.

Catalase is one of the primary enzymes measured in determining soil health. The catalase is given off by the microbes as they degrade organic matter (digesting their food) in the soil. Catalase is also used as a measure in waste and sewage clean-up. This enzyme is often present in these environments because it specializes in detoxification activities.

Some enzyme supplements include either catalase or SOD enzyme activities. Consider these ingredients as extra antioxidant power as well as potentially helpful with overall detoxification. It is not known at the moment exactly to what extent supplementing with these enzymes will directly benefit human health, although it is known that they are a naturally produced component of the body.

Lysozyme

Lysozyme is an enzyme found widely in plants and animals. It occurs naturally in milk, saliva, tears, and eggs, among other sources. The Paneth cells in the crypts of the villi produce lyzozyme in the small intestines. In the digestive tract, lysozyme acts as an antimicrobial agent working against certain types of bacteria by breaking down the polysaccharide walls of many kinds of bacteria. It also has some activity against harmful viruses and fungi. Thus, it provides some protection against infection and functions as part of the immune system. (Humphrey, Huang, and Klasing 2002; Gordon, Todd, and Cohn 1974; Imoto *et al* 1972)

Lysozyme is used as an anti-microbial preservative in some foods and pharmaceuticals, including throat lozenges and contact lens solutions. It is also available as part of some enzyme supplements. Lysozyme is also known as muramidase, and is commercially derived from the white part of hen's eggs. (Proctor and Cunningham 1988; Elison and Giehl 1991)

Immune system interactions

The immune system functions through a complex system of checks and balances to ensure that harmful substances are cleared from the body while the necessary 'good' tissues and organs are left to grow and function. However, sometimes this intricate system breaks down and the body starts attacking itself, or attacking normally beneficial substances in the body. Common autoimmune conditions include multiple sclerosis, chronic fatigue, fibromyalgia, cancer, and arthritis.

No one is completely sure what causes particular autoimmune diseases although a mixture of genetics, environment, lifestyle, and maybe even pathogens is involved. Currently, no cures for most autoimmune diseases exist. However, many good treatments are available, including enzymes, which allow you to live around the condition, and inhibit the situation from worsening.

A substantial amount of research finds there are compounds called circulating immune complexes that build up in autoimmune conditions. These complexes form when components of the immune system 'latch' onto or bind up any substance seen as an intruder in the body. More of these complexes develop in a leaky gut situation where improperly digested foods and toxins enter the body when they should actually be screened out. The immune system grabs the invading substance much like a policeman would handcuff himself to a crook so the crook cannot escape.

Under healthy conditions, these complexes are eliminated from the body immediately. In an unhealthy situation, these complexes persist in the body and may settle in different organs or tissues. Where these complexes accumulate may determine the type of symptoms you experience. For example, in arthritis, these complexes tend to settle in the joints. In multiple sclerosis, it may be the muscle or nerve tissue. In fibromyalgia, it may be the tissue surrounding the joints. Testing shows many people with autoimmune diseases have a greater number of these immune complexes, either lodged in tissue, in circulation, or both.

The accumulated immune complexes can cause inflammation, which is the source of much of the associated pain with these conditions. If inflammation persists, internal tissue is destroyed. These immune complexes can also contribute to cancers. Managing and controlling inflammation goes a long way towards limiting the damage caused by an autoimmune condition.

Proteases enzymes are very effective for controlling inflammation, and thus reducing pain and tissue damage. A multitude of research studies has shown that protease enzymes taken between meals sharply reduce pain and speed tissue healing.

So will getting rid of the all-important immune complexes help relieve the unpleasant symptoms? Research since the 1970s shows that, yes, eliminating these immune complexes improves many conditions including the ones listed here.

This begs the question, "How do we get rid of those immune complexes?" Digestive enzymes are one way to eliminate these problematic complexes. Enzymes work by breaking up the harmful complexes and activating macrophages. Macrophages are components of the immune system which gobble up and destroy the intruders. This ends the vicious cycle that leads to tissue deterioration and many chronic disorders. Certain mixtures of enzymes, including proteases, lipases, and amylases, have reduced the number of circulating immune complexes in studies such those reported by Stauder 1990, Stauder *et al* 1989, Ransberger *et al* 1988, and Targoni, Tary-Lehmann, and Lehmann 1999.

A problem with medications commonly used for autoimmune conditions is they often suppress the immune system. The logic is that since the immune system is waging the attack on the body, then suppressing the immune system reduces the problem. However, slowing or suppressing the immune system will also reduce the natural ability of the body to protect itself from invaders or other illnesses.

Autoimmune conditions such as Crohn's and ulcerative colitis have been hard to treat with currently available medicines. It is believed that the chronic inflammation involved in these conditions is triggered by immune complexes being deposited in intestinal tissue. However, German clinical studies show immune dysfunctions in these conditions might be effectively relieved with digestive enzymes that target the formation of these immune complexes.

The idea is to correct the autoimmune problem using enzyme therapy, not just treat symptoms. For these types of system-wide or 'systemic' uses, you should take digestive enzymes between meals, instead of with food. This permits the enzymes to be quickly absorbed into the body. You may need to experiment with several different enzyme products to find the one that works best for your situation.

Even if you start using digestive enzymes between meals you may see further benefit in autoimmune problems by also taking them with meals as well. This helps prevent the development of immune complexes before they can cause trouble.

In addition, taking enzymes with or without food can proactively assist in tissue healing. This characteristic of enzymes facilitates healing in a multitude of ways – preventing problems in the beginning, mending the root cause in the middle, and clearing out the toxins and debris at the end point. This all comes together to provide a system-wide solution.

CHAPTER 13

Viruses Part 1

– Guidelines for Viral Control

Understanding the viral problem

Viruses are both the bane and fascination of biology. Viruses are not technically living things, yet they require living things to reproduce. Viruses are particles made of proteins and DNA or RNA. Viruses are notoriously difficult to treat or control. However, digestive enzymes have an excellent history in the control of viruses. A number of references are given in the References section.

Viruses may enter the body by a variety of paths. An invading virus should be subdued and immobilized by the immune system, lying dormant and harmless in the body. In the gut, certain agents of the immune system in the mucosal lining usually conquer any viruses. However, if the intestinal mucosa is damaged or is deficient this can leave an opening for a virus to be reactivated, get out of control and become industrious in the gut, and even spread to other parts of the body. The same doorway results from having a weakened immune system. This may force the immune system to constantly work at a higher level. It becomes overburdened on a daily basis, yet cannot completely destroy or subdue the virus.

A number of research studies have established various viruses are present in some children with developmental delays such as autism, and often accompany persistent digestive and health problems. Documented viruses include the stealth virus, herpes virus, measles, chicken pox, Epstein-Barr, and viral encephalitis. There is evidence that viruses can cause dysfunction in the brain and damage the protective coating, called myelin, around the nerves. This leaves the nerves exposed and susceptible to damage. Viruses are suspected as agents in many autoimmune diseases as well.

A basic therapy against such viruses needs to focus on the immune system: improving its ability to function, strengthening it, and enabling it to work at a more typical rate and manner in addition to eliminating the pathogens, if possible.

Enzymes, particularly certain proteases, turn out to be an excellent therapy to use against a virus by working on several levels. Many viruses are surrounded by a protective protein film, something a protease enzyme may be able to break down. Eliminating this coating leaves the viruses unprotected and vulnerable to antivirals and destruction. Some virus coatings have carbohydrate and fat elements. Lipases and various carbohydrases may help disrupt the film a similar way. A few lipid based products having good antiviral properties are thought to work in this way (coconut oil, monolaurin, Lauricidin (TM)).

However, the main way enzymes may help in viral control is by working directly with the immune system. Substantial research shows how enzymes facilitate the immune system to work more effectively on health problems throughout the body in general.

Is there any evidence that any enzymes may be effective in the treatment of viruses? One example comes from a study by Dr. Billigmann. In 1995, he published the results of a study with enzyme therapy as an alternative in the treatment of the virus *Herpes zoster*. In a controlled study with 192 patients, one of the objectives was to confirm that enzyme therapy had been effective on this virus in a previous study. The other objective was to compare the effectiveness of enzymes with that of a standard drug called acyclovir. The high costs of treatment with this and similar drugs often meant patients with *Herpes zoster* would not receive medicinal therapy. The researchers concluded that overall the enzyme preparation showed identical efficacy with the drug acyclovir, and thus also confirmed the results of the prior study.

The *Herpes zoster* virus has been successfully dealt with since 1968 with enzymes. Enzymes are considered one of the best antiviral therapies with very few side-effects while also providing significant pain relief for the patient (Bartsch 1974; Scheef 1987). Bartsch eventually concluded it was unethical to treat patients with viral conditions with anything other than enzyme therapy because the enzymes proved far superior as a treatment.

Wobenzym also has clinical testing on some of their enzyme products with various viruses. This shows again that at least some blends of digestive enzymes can help with viruses for some individuals.

Besides the science part, or the theory, where something is 'thought' to work a certain way, I look at experience in real-life. The more the better. What I see after several years of working with the enzyme product ViraStop, looking into viral conditions, and talking to many people using ViraStop, is the results are basically that ViraStop is *incredibly effective!* People report excellent improvement with ViraStop even when other strong protease products at therapeutic doses did not help their chronic conditions or viral problems. Vitalzym is another product in this class of enzymes. I do not have personal experience with Vitalzym but others who take it report good results. This practical experience is consistent with past research results.

Less 'autistic' with fever

A special situation is frequently mentioned by parents of children with autism conditions. They note their child seems 'less autistic' when running a fever. Parents report their child's cognitive ability and communication drastically improve, and behavior is more typical. It is not known why this happens, or why it occurs only in some children. Perhaps this effect is more prevalant in those who have viral problems as a major factor contributing to their symptoms.

This may not be the fanciest explanation, but one possibility is that the fevers arise to fight off something harmful in the body. In these cases, that something might be a virus. Fevers often accompany viral infections. All enzymes increase their level of activity with increasing temperature until they get to a 'breaking point' when they are working so fast, and the electrons are vibrating so quickly the enzyme molecule essentially falls apart. It becomes defunct or is destroyed. This is why cooking or very high temperatures destroys enzymes. When the body runs a fever, it basically can stimulate its own internal enzymes to function faster, perhaps in an effort to overcome the harmful intruder.

Metabolic enzymes run all functions in the body, including the immune system. With increasing body temperature, the enzymes would be functioning at a higher rate (that is, they are working 'feverishly'). If the fever gets too high, the person suddenly dies, perhaps partly as the internal enzymes suddenly break down.

If a person is living with a persistent underlying virus, maybe which is causing the 'autistic' behaviors, a fever may be driving more immune system activity which then attacks the virus more aggressively. The viral load lessens, the person feels better and appears less 'autistic.'

Other symptoms or patterns associated with viruses are described in detail in the next chapter.

Virus control with enzymes
Related Symptoms
1. Have cycles or patterns of unexplained illness followed by spontaneous recovery.
2. Becomes more cognizant or 'with it' with a fever.
3. Never quite fully recovers following a viral illness.
4. Have repeated cold sores or herpes-derived mouth sores.

Viruses can be very stubborn. A program that has worked for many adults and children has been developed and is summarized on the next page. Feel free to adapt this to your situation, and chose among the various viral control measures. Updates and new discoveries in this area will be posted at www.enzymestuff.com and included in future printings of this book. Lab tests are available for different viruses. Consult your health practitioner.

What to Do Suggestions

• Start ViraStop (*Enzymedica; no other product has proven to give results comparable to this product at this time*) at two capsules per day between meals. If this brings an abrupt reaction, reduce it to one capsule. If the two capsules are well tolerated, increase the dose slowly by adding in one or two capsules per day between meals until you get to around 15 to 20 capsules a day. You may not end up needing that many, but it is a target number to shoot for. If one capsule of ViraStop is still too dramatic, shelve the ViraStop and use olive leaf extract (OLE) and vitamin C for several weeks. Then, restart the ViraStop, adding it in along with the OLE and vitamin C.

Some people see results right away. However, you may not see any change at all, not positive or negative, until you reach the therapeutic dose of around nine to 12 capsules. Experience shows it is common to see no change initially, and then when the therapeutic dose is reached, *bam!* you see abrupt signs of the effect.

Increase the dose of ViraStop slowly monitoring progress as you go. You may see drowsiness, a localized rash that quickly recedes, or other signs of viral control. Usually positive improvements occur at the same time. See the next chapter for specific results to look for.

You may notice a stair-step pattern where increases in dosage bring improvements that seem to fade away after a few days. In this situation, keep increasing the dose until the improvements 'stick' and do not fade. Consider this your Holding Point or upper dose. Keep giving this dosage for around three weeks. After three weeks, start reducing the dose by one or two capsules per day. The improvements should stay. If at any time there is regression, increase the enzyme dose back up a couple capsules and stay at this new dosing level for one more week. Then begin to reduce the number of capsules once again.

You may not experience this stair-step pattern. This is also common. If you do not see improvements fade away with increases in dosage (no stair-step pattern), continue increasing the ViraStop until you reach around 20 capsules per day. Usually a person sees more improvement with each increase in number of capsules. When you reach a level where there are no more improvements with dose increases, consider this dose your Holding Point. Keep at this level for three weeks and then start reducing the number of capsules per day as outlined previously.

Allow around two to three months for this entire process of slowly ramping up, the three weeks at the Holding Point, and then decreasing the dose. This is a very rough guide that is helping many people. Vary it as you see appropriate in your situation. If you are working with a health practitioner or doing other antiviral measures, you may need to adjust the time ranges because of synergistic effects between all the antiviral measures. Adding other antivirals tends to give better results than just enzymes alone.

Other measures for viral control:

• Olive leaf extract (OLE) - start slowly, give as is tolerated up to the recommended dose on the container

• Vitamin C - around 1,000 mg of vitamin C three times a day. Consider buffered C. It may be easier on the gut.

• Monolaurin or Lauricidin(TM) - coconut oil-based products with anti-viral properties. www.lauricidin.com

• Valtrex or Acyclovir - prescription medications for viruses may be offered by your health practitioner. These are not essential, but okay to take with the above measures.

• Lysine in the case of herpes simplex.

• Vitamin A in the case of measles.

CHAPTER 14

Viruses Part 2
– Results of Two Informal Studies

These trials were undertaken to see if certain enzymes thought to be beneficial for viral problems could benefit those with persistent viral problems. This was needed because other avenues, medications, and even other types of enzymes were not getting the job done, and families were looking for more options. This was a very basic evaluation to get preliminary information on the practical use of enzymes when there was a persistent viral problem. The results and accompanying research investigation yielded much helpful information.

Materials and methods

There were two main objectives. The first was to see if certain enzyme blends would help with viruses where other measures had failed. The second was to test the effectiveness of higher doses of enzymes. 'Higher doses' was defined to be more than the three to four capsules typically given of effective brands of enzymes. The research literature and anecdotal experience pointed to higher doses of enzymes being needed for more chronic conditions (such as cancer, pain, and autoimmune problems). Maybe doses of enzymes over and above the typical amounts of one to three capsules at three meals a day would bring a greater positive change.

The products in these trials were made by Enzymedica and tested independently of the company, although the company donated the product for these studies upon request. Volunteers offered their participation without compensation of any type other than receiving sufficient donated product for the trial. The investigating author (and author of this book) recieved no compensation.

The criteria requested that the participants needed to have a known virus (usually verified by lab tests). A few individuals had strong indication of a viral problem, including doctors' opinions, but no conclusive lab test identifying a particular virus. These cases are noted separately where appropriate.

The other main requirement was participants needed to already be using some brand of effective enzymes for food digestion. This was to distinguish any changes experienced with the trial enzymes from the regular benefits that can come from improved digestion with digestive enzymes.

The first trial was conducted with 20 volunteers who did not know what enzyme product they were testing. Participants were informed it was an all-protease product without any potential allergens, fillers, or fruit-derived enzymes (papain, bromelain, or actinidin which can cause problems for some individuals). This was to help the testing to be more objective. The enzymes were from off-the-shelf regular retail bottles and not something special from the manufacturer for this trial. Participants were told they did not need to change anything they were currently doing: therapies, supplements, medications, diets, etc. If they were already taking enzymes, they were to just add these new enzymes between meals on top of the regular supplement schedule. Participants could stop the trial at any time and for any reason.

Participants were to take the enzymes by starting slowly with one or two capsules per day taken anytime between meals, and then gradually increase the dose until they saw good results. They were to aim for around 20 capsules a day. This was to determine if higher doses of enzymes led to greater improvement. When asked, Enzymedica suggested nine to 12 capsules as the minimum for a 'therapeutic dose.' The 20 capsules per day was chosen because it was higher than what most people were giving, was above the therapeutic minimum, but below what is considered 'high' in other areas of enzyme therapy. In other areas of health, people commonly reported taking 45 to 90 capsules per day of various enzyme products.

Participants were to allow one to two months on average for this testing, and they could use as many enzymes as desired. Unlimited access to the product was offered so participants would not feel the need to ration their enzymes, and they would have the freedom to take more if the enzymes were helping.

Participants were asked for personal histories and to report any observed changes even if they were not sure of the cause of the change. Participants were asked to take detailed notes in a form most appropriate for their situation. A customized Nutrition Log was provided as one option for notes. Participants were asked to note any changes in eating, sleeping, bowel habits, behaviors, language, physical changes, cognitive changes, and any comments from teachers, friends, relatives, or other third parties. Participants were told this was new ground being explored, and any changes might be positive, negative, or no change whatsoever.

The first product tested was Purify by Enzymedica and was selected because of anecdotal reports of it being quite effective with viral problems. Some time after the first testing was completed, the formulation of Purify was refined, altered, and released under the new name ViraStop. Because of this product change, the second trial was undertaken to see if the results from the first trial could be repeated and were consistent with the first. Results could have been the same, better, or worse.

In the second testing with ViraStop and 21 subjects, the participants knew what product they were testing. They were sent full sealed bottles of off-the-shelf retail product as well as information from the first testing. Other than that, it was conducted in the same manner as the first trial. The age breakdown for both groups combined was as follows:

Age Range	Trial 1 (20 people)	Trial 2 (21 people)
0-5 yrs	6	5
6-12 yrs	9	10
12-20 yrs	2	2
above 20 yrs*	3	4

*These were adults with viral issues. Only one adult had a developmental delay diagnosis of ASD (autism spectrum). The other adults had suspected or confirmed viral problems, and most had autoimmune problems.

The reported viral problems were as follows:

Viral Problem (% of total participants)
Chicken pox/herpes	20%
Epstein-Barr	12%
Stealth	7%
Measles	5%
Multiple viruses diagnosed	41%
Unidentified suspected viral problem	15%

Results and discussion

In general, the results of both trials, first with Purify and then later with ViraStop, showed noticeable improvements for most participants. Since nothing like this had been undertaken before, very preliminary information and protocols were being worked out at the same time.

In both trials, the number of participants in any particular age group was not high enough to determine if one age group responded significantly better than another. However, there were individuals in each age group that did respond well. The number of participants with any particular viral problem was not high enough to determine if one type of virus was more affected than another. Nearly half the participants had multiple diagnosed viruses so determining the effect of the enzymes on individual viral types was not possible.

In both trials, degree of previous enzyme use did not appear to make a substantial difference. One person had been on three capsules of enzymes at all meals regularly for over a year and saw improvement with the addition of the Purify/ViraStop. Another person had taken enzymes off and on, one capsule per meal, and also saw improvement with the test enzymes. Most participants had used good quality enzymes with food daily for at least a year. This appears to show an additional 'anti-viral' effect separate from the benefit of enzymes for digestive health, and would be an area for more research.

In both trials, higher doses of 12 to 15 capsules per day seemed to make a bigger difference than fewer extra capsules. Some people saw improvement from the very beginning with just a few capsules. Others did not see any change at all until they reached 12 to 15 capsules a day at which time improvement began abruptly. There was not enough information collected in these trials to determine why some people saw gradual improvement in some cases with lower dosing, but others needed the higher doses to see any change. The differences may be related to the type of virus, individual differences in biology, or other health conditions.

In the first test with Purify, seven of the participants withdrew from the trial within the first month. This was due to several types of reactions which caused the parent to hesitate continuing the trial, although later these reactions were confirmed as rather typical of any viral control measure. In particular, a 'stair-step pattern' started to emerge and is discussed later in this text. Five of the participants had other issues come up in their lives (travel, other therapies, irregular dosing, etc.) and so the changes seen could not be attributed solely to the test enzymes or protocol. The remaining participants noted substantial improvements in several areas which will be discussed further in this text along with the results for the second trial.

In summary, although this first testing produced essential useful information, it was also compromised by being a pioneer effort with starts and stops along the way as the patterns and common reactions were being worked out. The second testing was much more consistent on several levels.

Using the guidelines worked out from the first testing, participants in the second trial ended up with an average dosing of 16 to 20 capsules per day of ViraStop between meals (the therapeutic dose). Two participants saw no change of any sort with this trial even at doses up to 20 to 25 capsules a day. However, these individuals had also not seen any change with any gastrointestinal or biomedical measure before. A couple of other people showed minor improvement with doses of 20 capsules per day. The parents expressed interest in using an even higher dose. It was suggested they increase to 25 capsules. At this dose, there was marked improvement and this was considered the upper dose limit for this testing.

Only two participants withdrew because the enzymes were not initially tolerated. Three participants had changes in their personal situations during the testing period. Because the patterns and reactions were better understood in this second testing, the families could better determine what was caused by the ViraStop and what was not.

Patterns and symptoms reported in these trials were checked against other types of virus control measures. The symptoms, or adjustment effects, which occurred during these trials were consistent with what has been observed with other effective antiviral programs.

Improvements observed

Improvement was generally seen in multiple areas of health and behavior at the same time. Even if there were some unwanted negative behaviors initially, there were positive improvements occurring at the same time. This is very consistent when introducing beneficial enzymes for some people during the initial weeks of adjustment. Improvements varied depending on the individual problems of each participant. The most notable and commonly reported improvements included:

1. Improved language and communication
Children having language or communication difficulties were reported to have improved speech and communication with others. This included being conversational, telling jokes, laughing with others, and expressing feelings and personal preferences calmly. A few people noted an increase in eye contact and attention from their child when speaking to him or her.

2. Happy Child Effect, less moodiness, better disposition
The Happy Child Effect is a term coined several years ago in the author's previous book. It describes a pronounced shift in the person's general disposition from being fussy, whiny, irritable, and argumentative to being cheerful, pleasant, agreeable, patient, and generally less moody. Little things no longer set the person off. Many people noticed the appearance of this effect and change to a much better overall disposition when reaching the higher doses of enzymes in these trials. Some people noted less anxiety in general.

3. More flexible in routine, better transitioning

A number of children became more flexible in their routine, had fewer tantrums, and could transition better between activities. Transitioning was done more cooperatively even with unplanned, unexpected changes.

4. Warts cleared up

At least seven participants noted that persistent warts on the hands or other body parts cleared up soon after starting the trial enzymes. Warts are viral in nature and this was a nice unexpected 'side-effect.'

5. Fewer cold sores, fevers, flu, and general illnesses

Most participants reported having fewer cold sores, fevers, flu, and other illnesses. Variations included not feeling 'run down' or continuously 'sickly.' One adult expressed it as simply finally feeling well. Several months after the trials ended, several of the participants continued to be free of being 'sickly' for unexplained reasons, and there was far less 'coming down with what's going around.' There were a couple reports of a child not needing to go to the nurse's office or staying home from school because they 'didn't feel well' or 'felt sick to their stomach.'

6. More energy (not hyperness)

Participants across all age groups expressed having more energy and less fatigue. This was not negative hyperness or out-of-control behavior. Children became more playful and easy-going while adults were able to be more productive by accomplishing typical physical and mental activities without strain.

7. More alert; cognitive improvement

Children were reported to be more alert and 'with it.' Cognitive improvement was noted as no more 'brain fog' or confusion. Reports included the participant was better able to stay 'on task' and showed an increased attention span. One specifically mentioned improvement in problem solving skills and memory. Some participants saw improved scores on school homework and class assignments. Others reported an expansion in interests (not just excessively fixated on a few).

8. Improved participation with others and socialization

Most reports included improved participation with family, therapies, schools, and peers. A few children were now playing with friends at recess instead of sitting off alone. A couple people said their participating child started playing with siblings, particulary when the higher enzyme doses were reached. Teachers reported the child interacting with others in class. This included cooperating in small group activities as well as verbally contributing to discussions. When it was time to be quiet in class, the child could behave appropriately.

9. Increased affection

One of the most blessed and welcome improvements was the spontaneous as well as reciprocated affection that many parents reported. Parents said their children became increasingly affectionate on their own, spontaneously giving hugs, cuddling, and saying 'I love you.' This was also expressed as genuine concern for others' feelings.

10. Decrease in sensory problems

Many parents reported that problematic sensory sensitivities dropped away as the higher doses were given. The child could better tolerate noisy or loud environments. Textures in food and clothing were much less a problem and the range of choices the person would accept expanded. Lights and colors that were previously a problem began to be much better tolerated and for longer periods of time. Children could better express they were uncomfortable in the situation without having a meltdown. This allowed the adult a chance to change the situation or take the child away from it.

11. Third parties commented on improvement

Several people reported teachers, friends, or relatives commenting on seeing improvements in the participant even when the person did not know about the enzyme trial. These objective comments help validate the improvements. The comments reported included seeing cognitive, physical, and behavioral improvements. A few reported therapists saying the therapy sessions had become much more productive and pleasant.

12. Adults reported substantial improvement in well-being

Adults' personal feedback differs from observing a child because an adult is better able to verbalize what they are experiencing. Several adult participants reported simply feeling substantially better overall, with much less fatigue and clearer thinking. One person said she felt she could do her job better and took less sick time from work. This, in her opinion, greatly contributed to much less stress and better quality of life. Throughout the feedback reports, the parents of participating children continually related how happy and relieved they were their child was doing better in multiple areas. In particular were the heartfelt thanks that the child appeared simply less miserable and much happier in life.

Summary of improvements

A general running theme that emerged was that the vague, unexplained feeling sick, drained of energy, and inability to think clearly that had plagued many of the participants for prolonged periods of time was significantly relieved over the course of these trials (via their own observations and reports). A few expressed they would be repeating their initial lab tests in the future to see if the previous viral measurements had decreased, but that has not been made available to the author at this time.

However, it was very evident that the trials resulted in real, noticeable improvements which were helping the participants in their everyday lives. And this was positively impacting the immediate family and people in the lives of the participants - a significant increase in quality of life.

Improvements were determined from feedback descriptions and based on observation by the individual adult or a child's parent. Approximate ranges for the level of overall improvement were used. Combined results from both trials follow:

No noticeable change*	10%
Mild but noticeable improvements**	26%
Moderate improvements	48%
Very significant improvements	16%

* Reflects no change of any type was noticed at the doses given within the time frame. This does not include participants who needed to withdraw due to other circumstances, although most of those had improvements to report as well.

**Several of the families in this group said they were proceeding slowly and never really got to the higher doses within the time allotted for this trial. They speculated the improvements may have been higher with higher doses or more time.

Ninety percent of participants completing the testing saw improvement of some type within the time frame. For three-fourths of that group, the improvement was moderate to very significant. The improvements continued after the ViraStop was discontinued. No difference was detected between the results of those having diagnosed viral problems and those feeling they had strong indications of a viral problem.

Other observations

About 60% of the participants noticed at least one of the adjustment effects described in the following text appearing at some point during the trial, if only briefly, and the rest observed no adjustment effects at all. Checking the research and anecdotal experience of several virus control measures, most of these are consistent with what is observed with any effective viral control measure. If any adjustment symptoms appeared, they were usually temporary, passed within a few days, and tended to appear soon after an increase in the Purify or ViraStop dosing.

Drowsiness

One effect noted in this testing was that participants would often experience drowsiness. This stood out because in the past years of monitored enzyme therapy with thousands of people, drowsiness had not been an adjustment effect or side-effect of enzymes. In fact, it is rarely an effect of any supplements. This was reported as the person sleeping more, drowsiness, and taking a nap when the person didn't routinely do so.

Stomach upset/flu-like symptoms

A few people found that taking the enzymes on an empty stomach caused some stomach upset in the very beginning. So they were told to go ahead and take the enzymes with food. The Enzymedica literature advises to take ViraStop with food instead of between meals if it initially causes an upset stomach. This solved the problem for those few cases and they still saw improvements. A few participants experienced mild temporary flu-like symptoms lasting a day or two at a time.

Immune system partner

The research literature contains very interesting information on the action of enzymes on viruses. When reading discussions on enzymes, note that the term 'enzymes' can at times refer to both the beneficial enzymes we take as supplements and the enzymes that are produced in our bodies. Other times the term enzyme refers to harmful enzymes produced by a pathogen. Viruses, bacteria, and yeast also make proteases/enzymes that can harm our bodies. This can be confusing unless you keep track of which type of enzyme is being discussed.

Proteases (the beneficial digestive enzyme kind) can enter the bloodstream and go about doing useful work. One of the ways proteases can act is to be preferentially connected to a component of the immune system called alpha-2-macroglobulin (written as A2M for short). The digestive protease enzyme and the A2M have a strong attraction for each other.

The protease connects to the A2M molecule and the A2M wraps around it, protecting the enzyme from being indiscriminately deactivated. The way this attachment between the A2M and the beneficial protease works is that the protease connects to a point in the A2M molecule just as it is attracted to any other substrate it can function on. But instead of breaking down the A2M molecule (digesting it), this action 'springs the trap' and the protease enzyme is caught. When the protease 'bites' the A2M molecule, the configuration of the A2M is physically changed, and the A2M molecule wraps around the protease. It sounds similar to an animal going for bait, springing a trap, and having a cage fall down on it.

In this cage, the beneficial enzyme is still functional. The protease is protected by the A2M yet still retains its activity. Similar to a caged animal still being very much able to eat, make noise, roam around and be active, yet it cannot escape nor can other animals reach it to harm or destroy it.

In addition, the A2M molecule appears to shuttle the beneficial protease to any part in the body that requires it. A2M sort of whisks the protease away to a site in the body that needs healing or is under attack. Similar to an emergency breaking out, an ambulance (A2M) is told to get any medical people (beneficial proteases) they can find. The ambulance goes to the places where there are medical people, and once the medical people are aboard, the vehicle speeds them off to wherever they are needed. Once at the site of the problem, the medical people go to work.

Research shows that when a beneficial protease connects to the A2M molecule, the A2M is switched from a 'slow' form to a 'fast' form. The fast form quickly mops up various compounds shown to be hazardous to health and disposes of them appropriately. This takes the harmful compounds out of circulation. The beneficial protease becomes a working part of the immune system to facilitate and improve function.

Viruses consist of proteins and have protein coats. Since the protease does not lose activity when combined with the A2M, it can still be effective on the viruses. This is an area research needs to explore further.

Many of the measures or medications used for autoimmune conditions aim to suppress the immune system because it is the immune system that is attacking the body. However, suppressing the immune system leaves the person open to more infections and problems as well as reducing its ability to fight off the virus. Because proteases work with the immune system, proteases can be used safely by those with autoimmune disorders. There is much written about enzymes assisting to control circulating immune complexes and how the complexes interact with the immune system.

Cycling patterns

An interesting pattern turned up as some of the participants were taking more capsules per day while increasing the dosing. The number of capsules would be increased and improvement would be seen. Then a few days later the improvements appeared to fade away. So the participant then increased the dose, and again more improvement was seen. However, after a few days to a week, the improvements would start to disappear. A stair-step pattern of increasing the dose and then having it slowly fade away continued. The overall level of improvement stayed above the starting point. I asked Enzymedica if they had heard about this because this was not a pattern seen with yeast, bacteria, or other problems. It was also not a characteristic of past experiences with taking enzymes. I was told, yes, this was a common pattern noted by customers.

This pattern might have something to do with viral activity and how a viral problem 'grows.' Viruses are elements that infect a cell. They are not true living organisms that are self-sustaining. Viruses have a totally different type of reproduction and infection cycle than bacteria, yeast, or parasites. Viruses manifest in a cyclical nature, rather than a linear or exponential pattern.

A virus attaches onto a cell. Then, the virus inserts its DNA or RNA into the cell using the cell's own resources to replicate many copies of itself inside the cell. This replication can happen in a short time, or over a long period of time. The virus may even hibernate or hide-out quietly in a cell for a prolonged time (latent over many, many years). At some point, the cell bursts open, killing the cell, and releasing the many copies of the virus which are then free to go out and infect other cells. The cycle continues.

Some parents have noted over the years their child may show a cycle of unexplained illness followed by spontaneous improvement. A parent would inquire why their child would be doing well for about six weeks at a time, then be really down and ill for no apparent reason and not responding to standard treatments. Then, the child would spontaneously just get better for another period of six weeks before inexplicably regressing again. This cycle would go on and on. The period might not be an interval of six weeks, but three months, four months, or six months at a time. It was the repeating pattern of unexplained getting ill or getting better that stood out rather than the exact period of time. This pattern has been speculated to be associated with a virus.

The cycling pattern seen in the person may be associated with the cycling nature of virus activity in some way (infect a cell for some time, explodes out in mass, infects more cells, followed by a latent period while the virus replicates inside of cells, burst out in mass, and so on). This pattern may be associated in some way with the stair-step pattern seen with enzymes used for viral problems.

The question, then, is how long do you continue to increase the enzymes throughout the cycles of improvements which then fade? The recommended pattern of dosing enzymes is to keep increasing the enzymes until this cycling stair-step pattern stabilizes. This is termed the Holding Point. Once at the Holding Point, continue the current dose of enzymes for about three weeks. Then, start gradually decreasing the enzymes. The improvements should continue and not fade away. If during the decrease in enzyme dose a point is reached where there is regression, increase the enzymes back up a notch for a week or so, and then try to decrease the enzymes again. It is the pattern that is more important than the specific numbers of capsules taken at specific times.

This strategy was worked out in the first testing and was recommended for participants seeing the stair-step pattern in the second testing. Only some people experience this, not everyone. Those following these guidelines reported success. Further evaluation of this will need to be worked out in future tests. However, these tests were quite valuable in bringing this issue to light, recording some preliminary information, and developing a general practical solution.

Viral rash and aches

A 'viral rash' is often reported as a characteristic response of any antiviral measure. This rash is noted with other over-the-counter supplements that affect viruses as well as antiviral prescription medications. The rash may show up right away or after a week or two of antiviral treatment, particularly if you work up to higher doses that begin seriously impacting the virus. This rash varies considerably by individual. Some people never see any rash, while others see a few spotty appearances of a rash, and others have a more pronounced temporary outbreak.

The rash spots tend to be very localized appearing on different parts of the body but they usually appear on one side of the torso or neck region, and go away shortly after appearing. It is common to see a small spot on one part of the body, and then later another spot in a very different location. It is not an all-over type of rash. The rash was usually reported not to itch, but in a few cases it was itchy.

One explanation found to explain this 'viral rash' came from experiences with other methods of viral control. The virus may be lurking inside nerve cells within the body. When being 'killed,' the virus can travel along the nerve endings until it reaches the surface of the body, or the skin layer. A rash may appear at the point of emergence. Sometimes this rash is painful or itchy, and sometimes it is painless. This is often observed as small areas on one side on the upper arms, torso, neck, or face.

Sometimes a person will experience muscle or joint pain when using an antiviral. The nerves under attack may also cause pain in the part of the body they connect to. You do not get an overall body rash or pain. You get highly localized aches or pain on just one side of the body (one side of face or torso, or one arm, or one leg, etc). You may also have milder muscle ache and no rash at all.

Note that a young child or person with communication difficulties might not be able to express this well. A child with physical discomfort may be extra fussy, resist physical activities, or have outbursts that are different than before.

In our testing, only a couple of people reported muscle or joint aches (it was not common under the parameters of the testing). If there is a viral rash, the rash might go away but any associated muscle or joint pain may linger a bit longer.

How long the ViraStop needs to be used will depend on the individual situation. Some people take longer to get to the upper dose or Holding Point while others get to that point in the first week. Some people may only see steady improvement with increased dosing and not the stair-step pattern. A timeframe of two to three months is reasonable if you are going to try this ViraStop format, although you may not need that long.

My experience with Purify

Right after the first trial with Purify and before the second one with ViraStop, I tried the higher doses of Purify even though I did not think I had a virus and was not feeling particularly bad. I did not expect anything to happen, actually. I had been taking enzymes for several years with meals, so I took 50 capsules of Purify a day: 10 capsules at a time, five times a day between meals.

About 48 hours later, I had a really painful rash on the top of my right shoulder. My arm *hurt*. It was not just an ouchy surface pain at the skin level. I mean it really **hurt** completely to the bone, much like I had seriously pulled every muscle in my shoulder. I could hardly lift a fork without my arm hurting. It was really odd. I did not connect this to the enzymes right away because I did not think I had a virus. And I was not hurting or in discomfort in any other way - no headaches, stomach ache, unusual fatigue, or pain anywhere else.

I stopped the Purify enzymes because I did not want to mess up my high dose experiment and thought that after a few days the rash would go away. The rash and pain stayed all week. It did not get one bit better even though I tried an array of topical creams for rashes and pain. The rash also did not spread or get worse (which is very unusual for typical skin rashes). Then I thought about the enzymes and started them again at 50 capsules a day. The rash started to go away and the pain lessened by half in about three to four days.

Then, I stopped the enzymes to see if the rash would just finally go away on its own (I was still not convinced it was viral). The rash stopped healing and did not get any better on its own for another week. It stayed at the very same level. After one week, I started the enzymes again (at 50 capsules a day). Then, the rash healed up completely. A mild lingering ache persisted for another two weeks before finally going away.

I do not know what virus it might have been but it certainly followed the antiviral control pattern . . . perhaps some latent virus. On the plus side, I found I was able to substantially reduce my daily migraine medication after the Purify without problem.

Combining antiviral products

Are enzymes more effective for viruses when used with other antiviral products or treatments or when used alone? Some participants were already using other measures for virus control. Participants were instructed not to change anything they were currently doing for these trials. The results from people testing various combinations of antivirals on their own since these trials show the combination of enzymes for viral problems and other antiviral measures tend to be more effective when used together. This synergistic interaction is consistent with that seen with both bacteria and yeast problems.

Post-test reports by individuals verified that, at least in some cases, this synergistic effect happened when ViraStop enzymes were combined with some other element with antiviral properties (Lauricidin (TM)), olive leaf extract, or a prescription medication such as Valtrex). Any other viral control measures available would also likely work toward the common goal of improving health against viral infection.

Alternatives for taking multiple capsules

Although the suggested higher-dose ViraStop program requires possibly taking quite a few capsules during the program timeframe, remember that this is only for a relatively short period of time of two to three months. This period includes the gradual increase in dosing in the beginning as well as the lowering of the dose at the end where you may be taking many less capsules per day. This suggested use of higher-doses of appropriate enzymes with viral problems is not a life-long program, or even prolonged over several years. Most of the volunteers expressed they had already been spending substantial time and money on other avenues without success.

However, some adults as well as young children may have difficulty taking so many enzymes each day due to swallowing difficulties. ViraStop enzymes can be taken by mixing in any food or drink. There is a list of mixing ideas at www.enzymestuff.com and in the author's previous enzyme books.

If cost or the quantity of capsules is an issue, some companies, including Enzymedica, offer more concentrated potency enzyme blends.

Please contact the enzyme company or a health care provider if this is of interest to you.

Conclusion

This effort was conducted to provide some guidelines and options for those who were looking for alternatives for virus therapy, and when other things had failed. For the past few years, successful guidelines had been developed for enzymes and bacteria problems, yeast problems, and sensitive digestive systems. However, there was still a great need for help with persistent viral problems. It was for this reason this pioneering effort was undertaken. The research literature strongly supported enzymes as part of a viral control program. In addition, there were already anecdotal reports of the Purify/ViraStop blend being beneficial with viral problems.

Since these trials were undertaken, many people have reported following these guidelines and general strategy with ViraStop with great success. The results, patterns, and symptoms reported have been very consistent with what was found in the testing. The symptoms of a stair-step pattern, spotty localized rashes, and drowsiness were included in some reports, but many people did not see any of these effects. Most participants experienced pronounced improvement in multiple areas of physical health, behavior, socialization, and cognitive improvement. These improvements remained when the high-dose ViraStop enzyme program was completed.

Whether any other enzyme products are capable of producing the same results with viral problems as found with ViraStop (Purify) has yet to be determined. Some of the participants in these trials had tried higher doses of other enzyme products previously without any success in this area. ViraStop is a unique special blend of enzymes that work together as a whole. Each type of enzyme has a very specific action. It is well-established that combinations of enzymes have pronounced effects in unique blends that the individual enzymes alone do not.

While these studies met their objectives, there are many questions yet to be answered in the area of enzymes and viruses. Hopefully this initial work will spur more refined research and add to the guidelines already found.

CHAPTER 15

Fiber

– A Diamond in the Roughage

"I have you now, Darth Mulch!" crowed Matthew swatting the mulch with his rake. Wood chips flew all around.

"Guys, could you just spread the mulch around right. Don't be so rough with it," I tried to sound serious through my snickers.

"You heard her," taunted the other brother, darting around swinging his rake like a lightsaber. "She said you can't use any force. The Force is not with you."

"Ha!" retorted Matthew. "That's an ol' Jedi mind trick. Or should I say, an Old Jedi Mom trick." He grinned playfully at me hoping for a good comeback. I didn't give in. Mainly because I couldn't think of anything snappy at that moment.

"Look, the sun's about down, so we need to finish up. What time is it anyway?" I asked while starting to collect the yard tools.

"A little on the dark side!" Two boys collapsed howling in laughter.

I sighed into the evening. That's it. Nothing productive is going to happen now. Might as well finish up tomorrow. I laughed at myself as well as with them. Was I really surprised?! The thought they would actually gain a better appreciation of nature through yard work must have come from a galaxy far, far away.

Foraging for answers

Soil benefits from fiber as much as people do. While not an exact correlation, mulch contributes to soil health in many ways, most not directly related to nutrition. The fibers in mulch consist of the hard-to-breakdown celluloses, hemicelluloses, and similar compounds.

Mulch keeps the tree and shrub roots insulated promoting plant health. It helps retain moisture so the need to water and fertilize is reduced. Mulch continually builds soil tilth. Tilth means the soil has better structure for retaining nutrients, water, root growth, and an optimal home for beneficial microbes and earthworms. Mulch smells and looks good - nothing wrong with a litte quality of life! However, the number one reason I am so fond of a thick layer of mulch is that in addition to all the rest, it controls the weeds. And I *really* do not like weeding. To me weeding is a major vortex soaking in time, energy, and even money.

So in essence, mulch helps control dysbiosis in the soil and among plants. In humans, fiber in the diet helps to control dysbiosis and disease in the intestines. Fiber helps to maintain moisture in the stool so it flows easily. Good digestive flow is necessary to keep debris and toxins passing out of the body. If you have bouts of diarrhea when ill, the right type of fiber helps prevent nutrients from slipping away too quickly. A different mix of fiber can also help constipation.

Fiber in the diet has been studied for some time. The health issues most commonly attributed to fiber include preventing and reducing problems associated with:

- Chronic constipation or diarrhea
- Coronary heart disease
- Bowel syndromes, diseases, and colon cancers
- Diabetes
- High cholesterol

Fiber is often mentioned as needed for good health, yet it can be a rather confusing subject. Much of the confusion comes from not understanding the difference in whether a source is referring to either soluble fiber or insoluble fiber. Although they are both 'fiber,' they function differently.

Soluble and insoluble fiber

Fiber consists of carbohydrates that are largely indigestible by humans, making it a poor source of nutrition or energy. However, it does have important functions in digestive health. The two main categories of fiber are soluble and insoluble. Both types of fiber form bulk and are important for good digestive health, although the two forms of fiber accomplish this in slightly different ways. The main difference between the two sources of fiber is how they interact with water and move through the digestive tract. Soluble fiber dissolves in water and forms into a gel-like consistency. Insoluble fiber absorbs water but does not dissolve or form a gel. The main features and benefits of soluble and insoluble fiber follow:

Soluble fiber:
- Absorbs liquid forming a gel consistency
- Delays transit time of digested contents through the intestines (helps correct diarrhea)
- Lowers total cholesterol and the 'bad' cholesterol - the LDL type
- Reduces the risk of heart disease
- Acts mainly in the small intestine and is then digested in the colon through bacterial action
- Thought to help regulate blood sugar which can be an important feature for those managing diabetes
- Sources high in soluble fiber include oats and oat bran, pysllium husk, nuts, flax seed, and some fruits and vegetables, such as apples, pears, berries, and legumes.

Insoluble fiber:
- Does not dissolve in liquid or form a gel
- Has no effect on serum cholesterol
- Speeds up the transit time of digested contents through the intestines (helps correct constipation)
- Poorly fermentable by colon microbes
- Moves bulk through the colon; helps regulate bowel movements
- Thought to help regulate pH in the intestines and inhibit harmful bacteria that could contribute to disease and cancers

- Sources of insoluble fiber include whole-grains, corn, flax seed (again), cucumber, and the skins of fruits and vegetables.

Most food sources of fiber contain some of both soluble and insoluble fiber, and not exclusively only one type. However, certain foods may be much higher in one type of fiber. Around 75% of dietary fiber in a typical healthy diet is insoluble and about 25% soluble fiber. Most people simply need to get more fiber in their diet overall rather than worry about the specific type of fiber they consume. However, to deal with specific health issues, focusing on one type versus the other may prove helpful.

With irritable bowel syndrome (IBS), the consistency of soluble fiber tends to be soothing and helps cushion severe colon contractions, whereas insoluble fiber and fats do not, and may even trigger sharp contractions. A diet lower in fats and higher in soluble fiber can be very beneficial in this case (in addition to enzymes, probiotics, and lots of water to go along with the fiber).

Soluble fiber tends to slow down the emptying of the stomach and digestion of carbohydrates. This may result in better glucose metabolism, which may help those with diabetes. Some patients using insulin are often able to reduce their insulin by following a high-fiber diet. Better regulation of blood sugar levels may help reduce hypoglycemic reactions.

Avoiding constipation is important in preventing waste and toxins from lingering in the body, not to mention helping one to feel more comfortable on a daily basis. When fiber interacts with water, it creates bulk. The bulk stimulates the walls of the bowels to contract, thereby promoting elimination. It may be helpful to note that in persons with neurological problems, this nerve-based feedback mechanism may not be functioning properly. In children and adults with neurological conditions, extra attention may be needed in this area because you cannot rely on the typical neurological response patterns.

In cases of encopresis, or chronic constipation, the bowel walls may be so stretched that the nerves are not triggered to send signals until the mass has reached an unacceptable size. This is why treating encopresis requires following a planned bathroom schedule for several months, even if you are giving proper amounts of fiber. Of course, adding fiber and the needed water will make the encopresis treatment proceed much better. Having sufficient fiber and liquid in the diet will also help prevent the encopresis problem from returning.

Diarrhea occurs most often only with a particular illness or event (such as eating a food you know you are sensitive to). Ensuring digested matter does not move too quickly through the intestines helps ensure your body absorbs vital nutrients from foods.

Soluble fiber binds with fatty substances. This may prevent harmful fats from entering the body, helping to reduce high cholesterol levels. It may also assist weight control diets. Soluble fiber can also help one feel fuller longer, and so reduce overeating. The exact mechanism by which fiber assists in reducing cholesterol is not well understood and thought to have multiple methods. (Howarth *et al* 2005)

In addition to binding with fats, the gel resulting from soluble fiber is able to bind with many types of toxins and debris. These unwanted substances are then carried out with the waste. If you are undertaking any type of detoxification program, ensure you have good waste elimination underway to quickly get the toxins out of the body. On the flip side, an excessive amount of soluble fiber can trap needed nutrients and inhibit digestive enzymes from reaching food for breakdown. So managing a balance to avoid too little or too much fiber is important to gain the health benefits of fiber.

The general recommended intake of fiber is around 25 to 30 grams per day or 15 grams of fiber per 1,000 calories. For children over two years old, aim for an amount equal to their age plus five grams per day. You may find more or less is needed on an individual basis. Eating about five servings of fruits and vegetables plus about six servings of whole-grains will usually meet these requirements. Most labels on packaged foods list the amounts and types of fiber per serving. However, too much fiber may interfere with the absorption of vitamins, minerals, and other nutrients. A daily intake of 50 to 60 grams of fiber is considered an upper limit. When looking at amounts of fiber, make sure to note if the amount is written as grams or milligrams. Fiber recommendations are in grams. It takes 1,000 milligrams to equal one gram of fiber.

Adding more fiber to your diet is best done by gradually increasing the amount of fiber over the course of a week or two so the digestive system can adapt to the change in diet. If fiber is increased too rapidly in the gut, a surge in probiotic growth can occur. Bacteria often give off gases as a by-product and any jump in growth can cause uncomfortable gas and bloating. One way to increase fiber quantities is to gradually substitute foods higher in fiber for ones you are currently eating that are low in fiber or low in nutrition over all (such as highly refined foods). To maintain bowel regularity, try to consume roughly the same amount of fiber all the time, and drink lots of fluids, including water, soup, broth, and juices. Just adding fiber without a proper amount of fluids can add to constipation woes.

If you make changes in your diet, you may significantly alter the amount of fiber you are consuming without realizing it. If a special diet focuses on carbohydrates in some way (high-carb, low-carb, adding or eliminating specific carbohydrate foods), pay attention to how this impacts your overall soluble and insoluble fiber intake balance. A major change in diet can come from a deliberate switch to begin a special diet, end a special diet, or add in previously eliminated foods once you start digestive enzymes. A slow change in eating patterns without thinking about it can shift the fiber balance as well.

Fiber-digesting enzymes - Friend or foe?

Most broad-spectrum digestive enzyme products contain some enzymes for digesting fiber. There are also special enzyme products that emphasize fiber-digesting enzymes. The enzyme products with the greatest amount of fiber-digesting enzymes are those for yeast control, vegetarian diets, diets high in fruits and vegetables, diets high in carbohydrates, and products targeting phenolic compounds. If you begin using one of these enzyme products, be aware that you may have noticeable changes in bowel patterns at least in the beginning because of how it affects overall digestive and fiber levels. You may need to eventually adjust the fiber content of your diet accordingly.

A common occurance when starting enzyme products with high quantities of fiber-digesting enzymes is that a person may think they have constipation because less waste is being eliminated. The key is to determine if it is true constipation where waste is being concentrated in the bowel making elimination difficult, or if it is simply less matter being eliminated. It is a well-known practice to give enzymes that breakdown fiber to livestock to reduce the amount of manure excreted.

Now consider the issue of fiber-targeting enzymes and fiber in the diet. Is it wise to take fiber digesting enzymes if fiber is so beneficial to health? This is an interesting question that would benefit from more research. At the moment, it appears that taking digestive enzymes is not a problem for dietary fiber.

Consider the example of mowing an overgrown lawn and letting the fibrous clippings fall back into the grass. A light mulch of clippings is beneficial to the lawn, a heavy mulch is not. When food is not sufficiently chewed and digested, it is like allowing a mulch that is too dense fall into the digestive tract. The dense layer of digested contents may be too cumbersome for any probiotics and enzymes in the gut to thoroughly break down. Adding some fiber-digesting enzymes enhances food breakdown so the fiber quantity is more appropriate for our gut environment. The idea is to ensure the fiber in the diet acts as an appropriate light mulch and not an excessively heavy mulch.

Taking enzymes may very well release any fiber-bound nutrients as well as the fiber itself from the rest of the food. If the fiber is bound within the whole-food, it is not available to provide its benefits. So in this way, the addition of fiber-digesting enzymes may be the missing key you need for your body to make full use of the fiber you eat.

Children with autism and ADHD conditions often have difficulty digesting fruits and vegetables because of food and chemical sensitivities. They miss the beneficial fiber and nutrients provided by those whole-food sources. These children are able to eat these foods when they start digestive enzyme products that are heavy in fiber-digesting enzymes (cellulases, xylanases, pectinases, hemicellulases, and so on). With the higher levels of fiber-digesting enzymes, they are able to get the fiber, nutrition, and other benefits from many fruits and vegetables, including antioxidants. Special products with high amounts of fiber-digesting enzymes may bring benefits that other enzyme supplements with 'typical' levels of fiber enzymes do not.

Consider a trial of an enzyme product high in fiber-digesting enzymes if your digestion and overall health is so poor that you are not able to get any benefit from the fiber in the foods you eat. If your digestion is fairly good, the fiber-digesting enzymes in a typical, good quality broad-spectrum product are probably sufficient. Enzyme products for yeast control also tend to be high in fiber-digesting enzymes. The enzymes work on the fiberous parts of yeast cells.

Let's say you have relatively good digestion, or are taking an amount of fiber-digesting enzymes that matches the fiber content in your diet. You may decide to add a fiber supplement to your whole-food diet. In general, it is probably best to avoid high cellulase and fiber-digesting enzymes at the same time as supplemental insoluble fiber. The enzymes may work on the insoluble fiber, speed its digestion, and may reduce its effectiveness. This is an issue with insoluble fiber rather than soluble fiber sources. Soluble forms work through dissolving anyway. Insoluble fiber goes through the digestive tract and has a type of physical cleaning effect, while soluble fiber absorbs water, reduces appetite, slows the conversion of carbohydrates to glucose, and binds with cholesterol.

Note: Enzymes can actually assist with most of the symptoms you take fiber for to begin with.

Keep in mind the benefits of both enzymes and fiber. The right balance of enzymes and fiber will vary depending on the situation.

Fiber - Food for probiotics

The beneficial bacteria in our intestines need fiber for food and fuel. The helpful prebiotics which promote probiotic growth (discussed in Chapter 10, Probiotic- Supplements) are non-digestible fiber. Even though humans can not naturally digest some types of fiber, bacteria can. Inulin and FOS are complex carbohydrates that can be found in certain foods or taken in higher quantities as supplements. The foods naturally highest in inulin and FOS are whole-grains, fruits, and vegetables. Notice these are also the food sources given for soluble and insoluble fiber.

Bacterial fermentation of fiber in the colon produces short-chain fatty acids which are thought to have an anti-inflammatory effect, may reduce insulin production, and improve lipid metabolism. In addition, the fermentation process alters the pH in the colon which inhibits the growth of harmful bacteria. One important short-chain fatty acid produced in the colon is butyrate. Research identified butyrate to be the preferred energy source of healthy colon wall cells.

Adequate amounts of fiber and water in the diet can promote probiotic health by preventing conditions which favor the growth of harmful bacteria. Constipation, anaerobic, and 'polluted' environments tend to promote the colonization of harmful species. Without appropriate fiber resources, probiotics cannot survive.

An area of current commercial and private research is in developing a category of prebiotic fibers known as resistant starches. Natural resistant starch produce more butyrate than other fibers in these studies.

And so it ends . . . and begins again

"Why do we have to keep putting down mulch every year?" Matthew asked the next day while he helped me finish the mulching job.

"Because it breaks down over the year and needs replacing."

"Why don't we put down rock like other people do. That way we only have to do it once?"

I am usually all for efficiency. The boys will be repeating my mantras on being efficient to their children and grandchildren much like I used to hear about kids having to walk five miles to school, in the snow, uphill both ways. Only my boys will be passing down sayings like 'It takes longer to do something over again than if you just do it right the first time.'

"Why did you volunteer to help me with the mulch?" I asked Matthew in answer to his question.

"Because the other two jobs you gave me to choose from were worse. I can finish this one the fastest and get more play-time," he answered. Free-time was golden to him.

Efficiency can be sort of like selective laziness. I just do not care to put out the energy to do something over if I do not have to. Sometimes that means putting in more effort up front to avert greater problems down the road. In this case, putting in effort to mulch and maintain a lawn means I do not have to put in far more energy later overhauling a weed problem, or dealing with poor soil. Mulch is a basic effort to promote healthy plants. Mulch keeps working throughout the year long after I have gone inside.

This love of efficiency is why enzymes appeal to me so much. Enzymes are so fundamental to health and they work at such a root level. I do not want to go back to chronic health problems or spend more money on medical bills, if I don't have to. Keeping up a basic enzyme supplement program and healthy diet saves a multitude of headaches down the road.

For me, I mean this literally. Taking enzymes means I am not losing over half my week to chronic migraines. It means my older son is no longer banging his head on the floor 10 to14 hours a day. It means he is not in a special education program, unable to interact with others around him. It means he has a reasonable future (of course, with his personal uniqueness tagged on). It means he has a life.

Maintaining good digestive health means my younger son can actually eat food properly and not lose the bulk of his childhood suffering with chronic digestive problems that would have affected his physical and mental development.

Getting rid of a chronic health problem is often accomplished much more efficiently and effectively with a core therapeutic enzyme program. Taking enzymes regularly means my husband's IBS and arthritis are no longer debilitating. Even if those problems do not disappear completely, the quality of his life has skyrocketed. I personally know a dozen people who have recovered from cancer and similar serious illnesses with the help of therapeutic enzyme programs.

It is hard to describe the joy of no longer living a life in chronic pain. The point where there is a galaxy of meaning in the reply, "I'm fine." They say a picture is worth a thousand words, but the real thing - the real experience - can be worth a thousand pictures. We may be at the end of our adventure with the major restoration of our health along with restoring the yard, but it is the beginning of the maintenance phase in both areas.

CHAPTER 16

Studying Stools

Stool characteristics and possible indications

Digestive enzymes may have a significant positive impact on regulating stools and elimination. A lot of information can be gathered from just observing stools. Color, texture, consistency, and other 'properties' can give clues to what is happening during digestion. Animal science experts and farmers have been judging the quality of manure for centuries.

This section is intended to help with stool detective work and is given only as a guide. Visually inspecting stools alone is not diagnostic of anything. There is some overlap in what stool characteristics may mean. Compare what you see as a stool inspector with other symptoms, behaviors, and tests to get an overall picture of what may be going on internally. Consult a health care professional with further concerns.

Also, what comes out one day may be due to something that happened on previous days because of the transit time in the gut. The evidence coming out one end may not be related to what went in the other end hours earlier in the day.

1. Black or tarry stools
Black or tarry stools (Melena) - the passage of black, tar-looking, and foul-smelling stools; can be an indication of digested blood in the

229

stool. Other causes are iron deficiency anemia, cirrhosis, colorectal cancer, disseminated intravascular coagulation, peptic ulcer, or stomach cancer. In advanced cirrhosis (liver disease), the abdomen becomes distended with fluid and ruptured blood vessels in the stomach and esophagus cause bleeding. The person may vomit blood or pass black stools. Very dark stools, for example, may indicate an ulcerative lesion in the higher digestive tract.

The ingestion of black licorice, lead, iron pills, Pepto-Bismol, or blueberries can all cause black stools or false melena. Stools should be tested for the presence of hidden blood if there is a concern.

2. Blood in the stool

Blood in the stool (Hematochezia) - the passage of red, or maroon-colored stools. Red or 'frank' blood in the stool could be caused by hemorrhoids. Bloody stools can also be seen in amebiasis, anal fissures, or colorectal cancer. Bright red bleeding with bowel movements may be due to hemorrhoids; however, other conditions such as colonic polyps or tumors, diverticulosis, and abnormal small vessels called AVMs also may cause bleeding. Rarely, the bleeding may come from the upper intestine or stomach. Blood, as seen in the stool, can originate anywhere along the intestinal tract. A black stool may mean the blood is coming from the upper part of the GI tract. At least 6 tablespoons (or 200 milliliters) of blood must have been lost in order to cause passage of melena. Maroon-colored stools or bright red blood usually suggest that the blood is coming from the large bowel or rectum. However, sometimes this can be caused by massive upper GI tract bleeding. Some upper GI causes of bloody stools can also cause vomiting of blood such as in peptic ulcer disease. Bleeding can be evaluated by colonoscopy. A definitive diagnosis will require radiographic and/or endoscopic investigation.

Black color:
- Bleeding ulcer
- Gastritis
- Esophageal varices
- A tear in the esophagus from violent vomiting

Maroon color:
- All the causes of black color stool
- Diverticular bleeding
- Vascular malformation
- Intestinal infection (such as bacterial enterocolitis)
- Inflammatory bowel disease
- Tumor
- Colon polyps or colon cancer

Bright red color:
- All the causes of black or maroon color stool
- Hemorrhoids
- Anal fissures ('cracks' or tears in the anal area)

3. Dark-colored stools

Dark-colored stools may be seen in platelet function disorders, iron deficiency anemia, cirrhosis, colorectal cancer, disseminated intravascular coagulation, peptic ulcer, or stomach cancer.

4. Gray, pale, putty, or clay-colored stools

Gray stools, pale stools, putty, or clay-colored stools can be associated with hepatitis, gallbladder disorders, or malabsorption conditions. Possible causes for clay-colored stools result from problems in the biliary system: the drainage system of the gallbladder, liver, and pancreas.

Bile salts in the stool excreted by the liver give it a normal brown color. Obstruction to bile flow out of the liver (cholestasis), or liver infections like viral hepatitis, may produce clay-colored stools.

Malabsorption problems or low bile output can cause undigested fat in the stool (steatorrhea) which is characterized by foul-smelling, light yellow to gray, greasy, or frothy stools.

5. Green, blue, or dark-colored stools

Green stools may be from bacteria, or a green or blue food eaten. Green, blue, or yellow artificial colorings can cause this too. Green stools can occur if you ate much more green vegetables than usual.

6. Orange-colored stools

Orange stools may be caused by certain medications. Beta-carotene (a form of vitamin A) may cause orange stools as a side effect so check any sources of vitamins or supplements, as well as intake of foods high in beta-carotene (carrots, sweet potatoes, etc.). Artificial food colorings, particularly orange or yellow, can also produce orange stools. If the stool is more pale-orange, a lack of bile salt (which gives stools a brownish color) is another possibility. Other sources are antacids containing aluminum hydroxide, barium from a recent barium enema test, and hepatitis. Consider checking some baseline liver tests to evaluate proper liver function.

7. Fatty stools (steatorrhea)

Heavy, fat-rich stools can indicate various intestinal and pancreatic disorders. This can also be caused by malabsorption or insufficient fat breakdown. Lack of lipase enzymes or bile output may be involved.

8. Diarrhea

Diarrhea is the rapid passage of stool. This is frequently considered to be three or more stools per day, or excessively watery and unformed stool. Chronic diarrhea occurs when loose or more frequent stools persist for longer than two weeks.

I generally think off diarrhea as the body trying to flush something out. In some cases the body may be trying to get rid of something it finds disagreeable. Or when the gut tissue is inflamed or damaged it is trying to get rid of irritants. When the tissue in the gut is not healthy, it may interpret otherwise acceptable substances as irritants and attempt to get rid of them by flushing them on through.

Diarrhea causes can be grouped into several general categories:

Pathogenic infections – viruses, bacteria, parasites, yeast. Pathogens can physically damage tissue directly. By-products or toxins produced by the pathogens can cause indirect damage and inflammation when they reach the body's tissues.

Food toxins - often referred to as 'food poisoning.' Toxins may be produced in foods as bacteria grow. This group of bacteria enters the body in contaminated food. These toxins are responsible for the vomiting and diarrhea associated with food poisoning.

Other non-food toxins may also enter with food or supplements. These may be artificial additives in foods, supplements, and medications (artificial colorings, flavorings, fillers, binders, extra synthetic ingredients) that are causing digestive distress.

Note: Some supplements or medications have enteric coatings. A commonly used older coating consisted of ingredients which could be irritating to the gut. A newer type of enteric coating is being used that is made from cellulose-type plant fiber. Some popular enzymes and probiotics feature this type of enteric coating. Be sure to check on the type of coating when you see the term 'enteric coating.'

Malabsorption - when the intestinal cells are damaged for any reason, they cannot absorb nutrients well, if at all. Poor absorption can also be caused by specific disease states, including: lactose intolerance, celiac disease (sprue), cystic fibrosis, allergies to specific foods, and pathogen infections. There are other causes of malabsorption as well.

Inflammatory Diseases of the Bowel – Crohn's disease, ulcerative colitis, and irritable bowel disease or syndrome.

Medications – antibiotics as well as other medications, chemotherapy, laxatives at doses too high.

Other - while the previous items are the most common causes of diarrhea, there can be other causes as well. Diarrhea can be a 'side-effect' or general symptom of many illnesses.

9. Floating stools

Stools that float are generally associated with some degree of malabsorption of foods or excessive flatus or gas. Floating stool is seen in a variety of different situations, the majority being diet-related or in association with episodes of diarrhea caused by an acute gastrointestinal infection. A change in dietary habits can lead to an increase in the amount of gas produced by bacteria in the gastrointestinal tract. Similarly, acute gastrointestinal infections can result in increased air or gas content from rapid movement of food through the gastrointestinal tract. One misconception is floating stools are always caused by an increase in the fat content of the stool. Increased air or gas levels in the stool make it less dense and allow it to float.

Another cause of floating stools is malabsorption. More than two weeks of diarrhea with floating stools is often seen in people suffering from malabsorption, a dysfunction in the gastrointestinal tract that affects the body's ability to digest and absorb fat and other food. Increased levels of nutrients in the stool (those not absorbed by the gut) are supplied to bacteria that live in the gut, which in turn produce more gas. This results in more air or gas-rich stool that floats. Note: the bacteria in the gut may be either the normal beneficial probiotic bacteria or harmful bacteria.

Dietary changes, diarrhea, and malabsorption can cause floating stools. Most causes are benign and will resolve when the infection ends or the bacteria in the gut become accustomed to the changes in your diet.

10. Stinky stools

Stinky stools - stools normally have an unpleasant odor, but one that is recognized as a fairly common or 'typical' stool smell. Stools that have an extremely foul, out- of-the-ordinary odor may be associated with certain medical conditions. Foul smelling stools may have normal causes, most notably diet. Foul smelling stools may occur in conjunction with floating stools. As you adjust to a new diet, the foul smell should return to the normal fragrant smell bowel movements tend to produce if just a change in diet is the cause.

If one of the other conditions causing floating stools is resolved, any foul smell associated should go away as well.

Sulfur smell - a few people noted that if they eat more sulfur containing foods and have a yeast problem, the yeast may feed on the sulfur foods and get worse. These cases also experienced an increase in yeast with sulfur supplements. Other supplements reported to produce a smell when not absorbed and metabolized well are selenium, glutathione, and SAMe.

If you have very sluggish digestion or constipation, this situation allows waste to rot in the gut to such an extent it produces this smell.

Extremely foul-smelling stools can be due to bacteria overgrowth. Some bacteria produce hydrogen sulfide which has a characteristic rotten egg smell (horrible stench). Ammonia smelling stools can be attributed to bacteria overgrowth or nitrogen being insufficiently digested or improperly metabolized. When food is insufficiently digested, the non-absorbed food can then become food for harmful bacteria or be putrefying in the gut. Either of these situations leads to toxins being released in the body.

There is an especially notable case which can occur with serious constipation problems. Bad bacteria can produce a stench so putrid, so foul, so horribly wicked, there is no mistaking it. This smell can be so horrendous you need to flee out of the house to get some air when the affected person is using the bathroom. This is a stench of such magnitude that your neighbors may come banging at your door demanding to know why you have a pile of skunks playing with stink bombs in your living room!

This odor is a dead giveaway there is a bad bacteria problem, usually in the colon. The person may also have bad body odor or bad breath, even shortly after a shower or after brushing teeth. If you have this stool stench along with chronic constipation, refer to the treatment in the next section - encopresis.

11. Yeasty stools

'Yeasty' stools indicate the presence of yeast overgrowth (such as *Candida*), but stool condition is not the only indication of yeast. Stools may appear during either yeast growth or die-off. Possible yeast-looking stools include:

- Cottage-cheese looking stool
- Yeasty smell to stools
- Stringy-ness to stools - like cheese strings
- Frothy stools - like when yeast cells are activated when making bread or when yeast bread rises

12. White specs in stools

- Rice (poorly digested)
- Been eating paper

- Consuming something else the body cannot break down. One person said this happens to her child whenever any kind of bean, nut, seed, grain, vegetable, popcorn, or similar was eaten.

13. Black specs in stools
Black specks may be seeds, foods, or from die off of yeast or bacteria. If you start any supplement that might create looser stools, temporary diarrhea, or die-off of yeast or bacteria (like an antibiotic, probiotic, digestive enzymes, antifungal, laxative, etc.), you might see dark or black flecks in stools during this 'cleaning out' period. Certain types of adverse bacteria in the colon can produce dark residues and this is being cleaned out.

14. Severe or chronic constipation, encopresis
Severe constipation, or alternating constipation and 'diarrhea' (or loose stools). This could be encopresis. More in next section.

Encopresis: What is it and what to do about it?

Encopresis is something to be aware of when there are possible intestinal health problems. It is more common than you might guess, especially in children. Encopresis can be thought of as constipation gone out of control. When the waste in the colon builds up for any number of reasons, you have constipation. If this is not relieved reasonably soon, the person can become impacted. An X-ray can show if there is impaction, if you want one done. At times, the solid waste builds up and causes the colon to expand to accommodate the growing mass. The colon can expand up to four times its typical size. Liquid waste may seep around the solid mass as well. This leads to streaking or staining in the underwear, smaller 'droppings' coming through, or what appears to be alternating constipation and diarrhea. Or constipation and a thick, pasty output. If you see any of these, consider encopresis and deal with it immediately because toxins may be stagnating in the colon and lead to even more problems.

The polluted environment in the colon may be killing off the beneficial bacteria and allowing an overgrowth of the harmful toxic bacteria. This can produce an incredibly strong smell. You may also notice strong body odor or bad breath even if the person just took a shower or recently brushed their teeth.

Indicators of encopresis are:

- Foul stools - we are talking knock-down hideous *stench*!!
- Foul body odor; bad breath - even after bathing or washing
- Chronic constipation leading to the elimination of massive stools (to the point they clog the toilet, and you are standing there wondering how that softball-sized mass physically came out of such a little kid?!)
- Leaking or streaking of stool in underwear; raisin-size droppings anywhere or everywhere
- Not being able to 'feel' when you need to go to the bathroom for bowel movement; also can manifest as a child wetting without feeling it

To treat encopresis, there are some options. If there is serious impaction, consult your medical care professional for ideas. The usual treatment suggests giving a laxative or enema to start breaking up the mass and eliminating it. Magnesium is a very natural route and works as a laxative at higher doses. Because magnesium deficiency is so common, this supplement might help with any additional magnesium needs at the same time. Some people opt to give one of the laxative products from the pharmacy or grocery store and use according to directions. Next, plan on keeping a very definite schedule of when the person goes to the bathroom to 'try' and see if anything comes out. The person should go to the bathroom about ten minutes after eating breakfast and dinner at least, and any other time after eating you can remember or it is convenient. The person should 'try' for about ten minutes long. This part is very, very essential to the program because it takes advantage of the body's natural digestive movements, and helps the body to get back into a proper elimination pattern.

It is common enough that the person may not be able to feel when they needed to go to the bathroom. They genuinely cannot feel the sensations. This may be due to the person having sensory integration dysfunction. When the person initially does not have the sensory feedback of when he needs to go, the constipation builds up, and then the problem perpetuates. Another route is that you may become constipated first, and as the colon stretches out, the nerves are no longer close to and in rhythm with the amount of waste. Even if the mass is eliminated, the colon is so stretched out it will not sense the build up of more waste until another massive amount accumulates. The problem again perpetuates itself. Scheduling times to 'try' is very important, because you cannot rely on the person feeling the need to go.

Adjust the diet to favor looser stools. Include more fiber and pure water. Many people also include something like mineral oil, commercial fiber products, or magnesium on a daily basis to keep things loose.

This anti-encopresis program needs to be kept up for a good six months or more. It is very common to see good results by the third or fourth month and to give it up because the person appears to be doing well. What happens is you may have re-established a good elimination pattern, but the colon has not yet contracted back to its original size. Some people are also very prone to becoming constipated and the situation can recur easily. So it is good to plan on six months or more.

If bacteria overgrowth has occurred you may want to consider a probiotic supplement at least for a while until the colon is normalized again. If the person has sensory integration issues, there are exercises available that can help regain better feeling in this area.

Using a natural antibiotic for the bacteria problem with constipation

For an 'antibiotic' for my son's chronic bacteria problem in the colon, I used Source Naturals Colloidal Silver. It comes in tasteless drops or a throat spray for about $10 a bottle. My son liked the throat spray. I did one spray in the morning and one at bedtime (half an adult dose). I did this for 10 days just like other antibiotics. I know some people say they use it every day or every week, but I am not comfortable using any 'antibiotic' like that.

It worked *brilliantly*! After years of horrendously stinky stools, the bacteria were gone. This was 'stinky' to the point the school was calling and saying he needed to leave the classroom because of foul stools and foul body odor (the boy bathed every day!). The colloidal silver was used after five months of many enzymes and probiotics -

nine protease enzymes and three Culturelle probiotics per day. The enzymes and probiotics helped noticeably but just couldn't lick the problem. The colloidal silver completely wiped it out. I do not know if I would have had such dramatic success with the silver without having used the enzymes and probiotics first, but this is just how I happened to do it. And we were plenty thankful to have such a cheap and easy solution after all those years. Some people are leery of the silver as it is a metal, so consider that. My son's bacteria was soooooo bad and sooooo long-standing, his health was deeply suffering from the bacteria as it was, so I opted for the silver treatment.

You might be able to use a prescription antibiotic or oregano. Those were not available to me at the time. I am happy to say that many people with a child in a similar situation have also had magnificent success with this treatment for this problem.

It did take a good four months of 'bathroom schedule' and magnesium before my son could really feel when he needed to go to the bathroom. So you do need to stick with the program a good six months. When researching the encopresis treatment, the warning was that most people see improvement by the third to fourth month and get lax on the treatment. And then the problem can easily develop again. Sticking with the program long enough for the colon to completely recover was important. My son still takes magnesium daily to keep regular. He just seems to have a sensitive gut. Our doctor diagnosed him with IBS at six years old.

If you have any questions on this, please ask. It is one of the most common topics I get asked about. Also, adults can have this problem too! It is particularly troublesome for elementary school age children. Adults really do not tolerate 'bathroom problems' in older kids like they do in preschoolers. An additional problem is the self-esteem issues that can accompany this problem in school-age children.

Using enzymes with constipation

When starting enzymes, some people think the child or they themselves becomes constipated. Please try to notice whether it is true constipation occurring or simply less waste passing out. This issue can come up with any enzymes, but particularly appears when fiber digesting enzymes are started. Fiber-digesting enzymes break down fibrous plant material (xylanases, cellulases, hemicellulases). Fiber-digesting enzyme products are usually those designed for vegetarian diets, or diets with lots of fruits, vegetables, and whole-grains.

In animal science, fiber-digesting enzymes are given to livestock to breakdown fibrous feeds, those with lots of roughage, so the animal can use the nutrition and energy from the food instead of it coming out the other end as manure. Producers do this to cut down on bacteria and toxins in the animal. This keeps the animal healthier as well as minimizes noxious odors. The reduced noxious odors benefit the animals and humans alike. These enzymes help prevent or eliminate colon problems in the animals. And on the very practical side, no one wants to shovel any more manure than they have to.

If you start enzymes, particularly fiber-digesting enzymes, you may very well see less material being excreted because more of what is eaten is actually used by the person. This is not true constipation.

Fiber with constipation

Fiber can be very, very helpful with constipation problems. Consider more fruits and vegetables, or a whole-food based fiber supplement. The idea is to add fiber which will absorb more water into the colon and help make stools softer and easier to pass. Insoluble fiber works best for constipation. However, *please* remember that the trick with getting fiber to work properly is to drink sufficient water along with the fiber. Lots of water. If you just pack more bulk into your system without sufficient liquid to move it along, you just add to the waste compaction problem. Fruits and vegetables have lots of water in them that you consume along with the food. This is why extra water may not be mentioned with those whole-food sources of fiber. But with other fiber supplements, drinking water keeps things loose and moving through your system.

CHAPTER 17

Troubleshooting Guide

If you started enzymes and interesting things happened, you may have new questions now. Also, the enzymes may have produced many improvements; however, there may be some behaviors or symptoms which are still unresolved - things that are left over. These leftovers can be quite helpful in pointing out what to look at next.

This troubleshooting guide presents some of the most common questions and issues that come up when starting enzymes, and how to deal with leftovers. It is important to look at symptoms as a whole because there is some overlap among all the possibilities. The suggested ideas to consider for each category are the streamlined 'best bet' practical measures that have tended to help the most people in that situation, not an all-inclusive list. Evaluate each in light of your own situation. It is suggested to do each recommended item one at a time, and not all of the suggestions the same day. Starting one thing at a time will help you determine if that one thing is helping and if you even need to go on to something else.

Situation 1. Some foods still need to be eliminated even after taking enzymes for several weeks

Related Symptoms

1. Inconsistent results with enzymes.
2. Different reactions when eating in different places (ex. home, restaurant).

You may have had many food intolerances and starting good quality digestive enzymes allowed nearly all foods to be reintroduced except for a few. You may be wondering, 'Why did enzymes help with other foods but not these few?' When certain foods cannot be added back into the diet but many others can, a good place to start is to look at what is common among these excluded foods. There may be a shared chemical compound or physical structure involved. For example, if the only food not covered by enzymes is the group bananas, oranges, and tomatoes, consider amines as a possible problem.

If you can now eat cheeses but not drink milk, consider what may be in the milk product that is not in the cheese form of dairy. If you drink low-fat milk, consider there may be a hidden artificial preservative in the vitamin A which was added to the milk. To test this, try whole milk for a week and see if there is any improvement. If so, you know that 'dairy' foods are not the actual problem, something else is.

What to do suggestions

- Write down foods that cannot be eaten.
- Write down any foods in that same category that can be eaten
  examples:
    food category is dairy: cheeses - yes, milk -no
    food category is fruits: pears - yes; raisins - no
    food category is gluten: homemade bread - yes, store bread - no

- Investigate what is different about the foods that cannot be eaten from other foods in the same food category. (your reference A)

- Investigate what is similar about the foods that cannot be eaten. (your reference B)

- Working simultaneously with your reference lists A and B may help you find a common denominator to target the problem

Situation 2. The main problem foods are bananas, tomatoes, and oranges after taking enzymes for several weeks

Related Symptoms
1. Problems sleeping, either getting to sleep or staying asleep.
2. Irritability, moodiness, anxiety, poor attention, fidgety, jumpy.
3. Frequent histamine reactions; reacts to 'everything.'

A common chemical denominator among these foods is they are all high amine foods. Consider amines may be an issue, especially if other fruits and vegetables can be eaten without problem. Serotonin is an amine compound that leads to the formation of melatonin, an amine needed for proper sleep. Poor amine processing can result in low serotonin problems and poor sleep. Serotonin is also a factor in good, even mood. Allergies involve histamine reactions. Hist*amine* is an amine by definition. When histamine processing is off in the body, or histamine levels run high, you can experience oddball histamine or allergic reactions to many compounds as the body is overreacting to everything.

If you experience most of this set of reactions, the problem may involve inappropriate amine use by the body (something enzymes do not affect directly) instead of amines not being freed from food (something enzymes affect directly). These reactions may go away after more gut healing occurs, and the serotonin receptors are functioning better. Healing the gut also reduces the amount of compounds leading to histamine reactions.

What to do suggestions

- Epsom salts - either as a bath, lotion, or skin wash.

- Antioxidant supplements for detoxification, such as vitamin C.

- Look up other high histamine foods and chemicals, and reduce or avoid those for awhile. Histamine foods/chemicals are also a known migraine trigger.

- Watch your protein intake initially to reduce excess amines in the system. *see Hypoglycemia, page 246*

Situation 3. Problems with hypoglycemia

Related Symptoms
1. Has *Candida* yeast or problem bacteria.
2. Irregular eating habits; does not eat at regular intervals.
3. Craves or eats lots of simple carbs, sugary foods, processed foods.
4. Prone to significant unexplained mood swings in the same day.

Hypoglycemia can really mess with your head and energy levels. These problems result from large swings in blood sugar levels. A highly sensitive person, or person with neurological issues, is more sensitive to these ups and downs. What is a negligible change for one person can send another into a tailspin. People with yeast overgrowth usually have hypoglycemia problems.

The problems from hypoglycemia can be drastically reduced by following some simple eating management practices. The idea is to eat so blood sugar levels remain as steady as possible. The type of food combinations as well as frequent eating helps food to be digested and absorbed into the body at a more constant rate. This leads to more even blood sugar levels.

A glycemic index rates how quickly foods are digested and to the degree they affect blood sugar. Some current diets revolve around the glycemic index. Glycemic indexes are available through most dieticians, and there are some links at www.enzymestuff.com.

What to do suggestions

- Eat at least six times a day; eat something every 3 to 4 hours.

- Eat a wholesome complex carbohydrate food with a protein food at each meal or snack. (can be as simple as peanut butter and crackers or apple; cheese on celery sticks)

- Review a glycemic index to learn food digestion rates.

- Take a good quality broad-spectrum enzyme with meals.

- Increase soluble fiber with meals.

Situation 4. Inconsistent results - enzymes appear to work some of the time but not other times

Enzymes work on contact, so it could be they are not consistently in contact with the foods they need to work on. Inconsistent or poor results are often resolved by swallowing the capsules earlier to ensure there is time for the enzymes to be released from the capsules, particularly if the enzymes are in vegetable-based capsules (most are). This is usually not an issue with fairly healthy digestion (the type of conditions laboratories typically design capsules for). However, those with impaired digestion tend not to have the 'standard' healthy digestive conditions, so capsules may not be dissolving quickly enough.

Opening capsules and mixing the enzymes in a food or drink, using a bulk powder, or a chewable enzyme may give better results because it ensures the enzymes are out of the capsule and in contact with the food.

In the beginning especially, some people get best results when giving enzymes at all meals and snacks. Any food may be triggering adverse reactions initially, particularly with a leaky gut situation.

A higher dose of enzymes may be needed for consistent results. If you find higher doses are needed, you may want to switch to a more therapeutic enzyme product, or one with greater enzyme activity.

What to do suggestions

- If swallowing capsules, take 20 to 30 minutes before eating. Or open capsules and mix enzymes in a bite of food or drink.

- Give enzymes at all meals and snacks for one week and see if this gives more consistent results.

- Increase the dose of enzymes for several days and see if this gives more consistent results.

- Check if there is a food or chemical that is eaten when the enzymes appear not to work that is not present when the enzymes appear to work. The food or chemical may be masking the improvements with enzymes. *see page 244*

Situation 5. Do not see any results with enzymes, or very poor results

See Four possible reaction patterns, page 86, for discussion on results.

What to do suggestions

- If you know you have a yeast or bacteria overgrowth, you can expect to see more reactions from die-off. The negatives caused by die-off may mask any improvements initially, and positive results may take a little longer to see. Yeast or bacteria flare-ups tend to mask the benefits the enzymes are providing. If you have yeast or bacteria issues, know that you may need to allow a little longer than the initial few weeks for adjustment.

- A chronic toxic burden in your body may cloud improvements with enzymes. Some people who saw no results at all with enzymes then went on to start a detoxification program (even if it was just judicious doses of antioxidants). After some detoxification, they then saw improvement with enzymes. Keep in mind that enzymes themselves can help relieve the toxin burden on the body. Enzymes can be a great part of a cleansing program.

- Check if there may be a food or chemical in the diet, body care items, or environement that needs to be removed and is masking other improvements. In particular, enzymes may not help with a true allergy (such as a peanut or shellfish allergy) or intolerance to nuts. Enzymes tend not to help with artificial colorings, flavorings, preservatives, or other additives (such as sulfites, benzoates, etc). Colorings are common on medications so you can readily tell them apart. You may be able to wash this coloring off, or you can ask for the medication to be compounded without artificial coloring or flavorings.

- Reaction to product formulation - Some people may react negatively to something in a particular formulation. Check the product to see if any of the fillers or additives may be a problem.

more . . .

A common problem, particularly with children having hyperactivity disorder or behavior problems, is an intolerance to the fruit-derived enzymes (bromelain, papain, actinidin, and ficin). If the child has known negative behavior problems, try an enzyme product without these fruit-derived enzymes. It is also possible that a person will react to a particular mixture as a whole and no specific item is identified as the offender.

• At times, the particular enzyme formulation you are taking is not appropriate for your needs. Even if it is targeting the goals you want, you may get better results with a different brand or formulation. Even if the labels seem rather similar, you may get notably better results from one product over another due subtle enzyme interactions among the different blends. Many manufacturers will send you samples upon request.

• If the person is older, allow more time, up to two to three months. Most older people see improvement immediately, but some show improvement on a more slow yet steady progression.

• Try increasing the dose of the enzymes for a few days. It could be you need more enzymes initially to see a change, or that the chosen product has lower enzyme activity. Taking as much as five to eight capsules per meal should be enough to tell if you need higher concentrations of enzymes. If higher doses do initiate a change, you can either give higher amounts of your chosen product, or start investigating another product that has higher levels of enzyme activity per capsule.

• If no reaction at all is seen by the third or fourth week, neither positive nor negative, and you have accounted for all the previous items, then it is up to the individual whether to continue with enzymes or not. The enzymes might be working well behind the scenes but is just not visibly evident. Continuing enzymes while pursuing other avenues has many advantages. Enzymes will help the gut stay in better condition, improve nutrition, and better support the body while you are implementing other measures to improve health. However, it is also hard to justify spending time and money on an avenue that is not producing visible results.

Situation 6. Hyperactivity - positive or negative

Related Symptoms
1. Positive hyperactivity - general good mood; very active; may be chatty; excess energy; very 'awake' and alert.
2. Negative hyperactivity - general bad mood; irritable; fussy; picking fights; pestering others; headache or feeling sick; destructive behavior.

There are several reasons a person may exhibit hyperactivity in the very beginning with enzymes. The most common reasons follow.

1. Hyperactivity may be a reaction from sudden withdrawal from a food, usually a carbohydrate or sugar, or other substance that is now being properly broken down with enzymes. This can happen even though you may already have been on a restrictive diet for these foods, or you have sharply reduced them from your diet.

2. The person taking enzymes may be trying to adjust to an increase in awareness or sensory input (such as lights, sound, motion, textures, smells). It can also be an adjustment to sensing the world differently than before. Improvement may also bring an increase in stimming, hyperactivity, anxiety, and a bit of sound sensitivity as the person adjusts to processing and interpreting a different level of sensory input and stimuli. *see pages 77-78*

3. Enzymes are known to help keep yeast and bacteria in check. You may see a temporary increase in bowel movements, irritability, flu-like symptoms, hyperactivity, or a change in appetite during this die-off period just as you do with other pathogen control efforts.

4. Better digestion and overall improvement in health with enzymes may unmask a nutrient deficiency. A common deficiency is magnesium. Symptoms of magnesium deficiency are hyperactivity, anxiety, and muscle spasms. Adding a soluble form of magnesium may be very helpful. Magnesium has no known toxic levels and is inexpensive. *see Magnesium, page 264*

5. If you are only taking a protease enzyme product, one that breaks down only proteins, an influx of amino acids into the system may

more . . .

cause hyperactivity. Amino acids tend to be stimulatory in nature. If you are taking amino acid supplements, the enzymes may be facilitating more absorption of the supplement resulting in hyperness. Similar to the type of 'up' or jittery feeling high-protein/low-carbohydrate diets can produce. Balancing the amino acids with more carbohydrates may help in this situation.

6. A particular food may still need to be eliminated. Artificial additives, phenolic compounds, and excess amines tend to cause hyperness and poor sleep. These may need to be reduced from the diet even with enzymes. Epsom salt baths (magnesium sulfate) tend to be very helpful in reducing these adverse effects. Epsom salts supply two ingredients, magnesium and sulfur, in readily bioavailable forms that can help to process out these compounds.

What to do suggestions

- Determine if it is positive or negative hyperactivity.

- If positive, provide more activities, both mentally and physically allowing the person time to adjust to changes. Alternately, a person may need more breaks or less activity for awhile.

- If negative, check if there are any positive improvements happening at the same time. Any positives at all. If so, the negatives are usually part of the typical adjustments and will fade within one day to three or four weeks.

- If negative, determine if it could be bacteria, yeast, or viral die-off, or withdrawal from certain foods.

- Reduce the dose of enzymes if the negatives are too uncomfortable. Reduce any high protease enzyme product, or stop it for about a week before starting again at a lower amount. see *The Great Low-n-Slow Method, Chapter 6*

- Give Epsom salts and magnesium to help with calming. Magnesium is very often deficient. Choose a soluble form (not magnesium oxide). see *Magnesium, page 264*

- Balance a high protein intake with more carbohydrates.

Situation 7. Negative hyperactivity

Related Symptoms
1. Poor sleeping, either getting to sleep or staying asleep.
2. Eats a diet high in highly processed foods.

Hyperactivity may be described as either positive or negative. Positive hyperactivity means the person has lots of energy and is always go, go, go. However, the person's mood is usually upbeat and the hyperactivity can be channeled into constructive activities. For this type of hyperactive child, playing outside, physical activity, or more activities of any kind can work out nicely. Adults can usually realize they have more energy, and are 'up.' It is not unusual to feel a little strange at this newfound energy for a few days or weeks until you adjust.

Negative hyperactivity describes a person who is fussy, irritable, picking arguments, and overall in a disagreeable mood. Children may be distructive, antagonistic, and hurtful to others or themselves. Alternately, they may be emotionally fragile or cry easily.

It is the negative hyperactivity that may be related to a nutritional problem. If one of the nutritional changes does not resolve the problem, consider other non-nutritional avenues such as sensory triggers or more intense physiological problems. Negative hyperactivity is also associated with die-off or viral control if you are using something to control pathogens.

What to do suggestions

- Epsom salts - either as a bath, lotion, or skin wash.

- Magnesium supplements - a well-absorbed form, not oxide
  see Magnesium, page 264

- Amines, sulfites, nitrites, and nitrates may cause this negative reactions. see page 254

more . . .

- Artificial additives, including in supplements and medications, tend to cause problems for this group in particular. Some artificial colorings on medications will wash off with water. Otherwise you can ask for the medication to be compounded without artificial coloring.

- Consider sources of compounds known as salicylates or phenols. Phenols occur throughout nature and are often the healthful antioxidants needed for good detoxification in the body. However, people with negative hyperactivity tend to have a problem processing these phenol compounds appropriately. Eliminating sources of high phenols is one option. However these are often the highly colored fruits and vegetables known to be effective antioxidants and excellent for good health.

- Look into the Feingold Program and Failsafe Program. These nutritional programs focus on identifying various compounds in foods and body care products, both naturally occurring and artificial. The Failsafe Program focuses on a much wider range of compounds. Both programs list research studies on many of these compounds as resources:

  www.fedupwithfoodadditives.info
  www.feingold.org

- Fiber digesting enzymes tend to help this group greatly. Taking good quality fiber digesting enzymes appears to breakdown the foods so the phenols can be used for good health and not cause a problem. Look for products such as V-Gest or any of the main enzyme products used with yeast control: Candidase, Candizyme, Candex. see *Enzymes for Yeast, page 160*

- If this sort of behavior arises when undertaking a pathogen control or detoxification effort, such reactions can be part of the 'house-cleaning' process. Consider some of the measures listed on page 174 to manage die-off.

Situation 8. Child shows super-nasty, defiant attitude

Related Symptoms
1. Tends to occur most in boys, but does not occur all the time.
2. May have negative hyperactivity and other behavior issues.

This antagonistic mood tends to be characteristic with sulfite and nitrite intolerances. The body converts sulfur to sulfite and then to sulfate. Some people have problems with the conversion step of sulfur to sulfite. Others have problems with the step converting sulfite to sulfate.

$$\text{sulfur} \xrightarrow{\ 1\ } \text{sulfite} \xrightarrow{\ 2\ } \text{sulfate}$$

MSM is a supplement with sulfur in the form of sulfite. If you have trouble with the first conversion step, MSM should be helpful. However, if you have trouble with the second conversion step, you would still have difficulty processing MSM. Epsom salts contains sulfur in the form of sulfate (no more conversion is necessary). If you do not tolerate MSM but do fine with Epsom salts, this may indicate an issue with the second step in the conversion pathway. If you get great results from MSM, then the second step is likely not a problem, but the first step is.

What to do suggestions

- Avoid sources of naturally occuring sulfites, nitrates, and nitrites. One may be a problem source, while another is not. Epsom salts are magnesium sulfate and tend to be quite helpful for this problem. Nitrites are often in preserved meats (including in lunch meats, pizza, and meats in the meat counter). Sulfites are often in fruit juices and carbonated drinks.

- Epsom salts - either as a bath, lotion, or skin wash.

- Magnesium supplements - a well-absorbed form, not oxide
  see Magnesium, page 264

Situation 9. Poor sleep

Related Symptoms
1. Hyperactivity or sluggish fatigue.
2. Moodiness, irritability, depression, anxiety.
3. Sensory integration problems.
4. Yeast or bacteria problems.
5. Head-banging, physical self-destructive behavior.
6. Amine intolerance, protein intolerance.

Sleep is essential for proper neurological function. Any typical person functions poorly when constantly sleep-deprived. Poor sleep includes disrupted sleep, not enough sleep, difficulty in getting to sleep, and getting good quality sleep. Poor sleep affects sensory processing and the interpretation of pain. It also affects cognitive ability and mood. If sleep is a problem, fixing the sleep situation may go a long way toward resolving behavioral, cognitive, and physical problems. There are many reasons for poor sleep and only some basic ideas are given here.

What to do suggestions

- Protease enzymes for thorough digestion of proteins. Balance high protein diet with complex carbohydrates. Check for amine intolerance. *see amines, page 245*

- Epsom salts, magnesium and sulfate. Check for magnesium deficiency. *see Magnesium, page 264*

- Consider melatonin supplements. Usually sold in 1 to 3 mg. amounts. Medications for sleep or pain, such as amitryptiline, may be helpful. Short-term use may be enough to re-regulate the sleep cycle, or until other root problems can be corrected.

- Reduce sensory stimulation throughout the day and especially in the evening for sensitive people. Establish a sleep preparation routine and good sleep environment. Something as simple as having the right texture and weight of pajamas and bedding can make all the difference for a highly sensitive person.

- Serotonin imbalance. *see page 256*

Situation 10. Tryptophan, 5-HTP supplements, and SSRI medications

Related Symptoms
1. May have sleep problems.
2. Moodiness, anxiety.
3. Trouble digesting meats; poor reaction to amino acid supplements.
4. Carbohydrate or dairy cravings.

The amino acid tryptophan is first converted to 5-HTP. 5-HTP is eventually converted to serotonin, the important neurotransmitter involved in proper sleep, pain control, mood regulation, and inhibiting obsessive tendencies and aggression. Foods that tend to boost tryptophan are bananas, dairy, whole grains, and turkey. If your body is not getting enough serotonin, you may crave these foods.

Taking tryptophan or 5-HTP supplements work to increase the total amount of serotonin in the body. Some of the total amount of trytophan goes into forming serotonin and the rest goes to other tryptophan needs, such as producing proteins. 5-HTP is not shuttled off for these other uses. These two supplements as well as whole-foods add more serotonin into the body.

Selective serotonin reuptake inhibitors (SSRIs) are a class of medications that work by forcing the body to reuse whatever quantity of serotonin is available in the body. SSRIs do not add more serotonin, they help the body get more use out of, or use more efficiently, whatever serotonin is present.

If someone runs high in serotonin anyway, and they take an SSRI, they tend to get much worse because they already have excess serotonin to begin with. If the person is too low in serotonin, they will likely benefit from an SSRI. If the person already has average levels in serotonin, the medication may not do anything or possibly make them worse as the medication pushes the 'adequate' level into the 'high' range. I have experienced being way too high in serotonin and way low. Both extremes are unpleasant.

Making sure the supply of tryptophan is adequate may be a better first step because tryptophan is used in other places in the body.

more . . .

Correcting a tryptophan deficiency may help clear up other tryptophan-associated problems. Then if additional tryptophan input does not resolve the problem, try 5-HTP. If that does not resolve the problem, consider an SSRI. Different people respond best to each of these options depending on where the glitch in their serotonin use pathway is.

Note: since most of the serotonin action is located in the gut, if you have a damaged gut, you are quite likely to also have disrupted serotonin. As the gut heals, the serotonin processing cells form and function properly, and these problems may lessen or go away. (Bearcroft, Perrett, and Farthing 1998; Jaffe 1990; Wood *et al* 1999)

Personal experience:

My family responds quite well with SSRIs. Zoloft works best for us. I tried 5-HTP a couple times, but just could not get it to produce consistent results. I could not find a 'stable' dose. I could tell the 5-HTP was doing something, because the adjustment effects from the 5-HTP were the same as for the medication for me. But my results kept bouncing all around with the 5-HTP. In the end, I went back to the Zoloft because the results were quite stable and even. Apparently my particular problem responded best by the medication working on the efficient *use* of serotonin, and not by the supplement working on increasing the overall *supply* of serotonin.

What to do suggestions

- Adjust the diet to favor more trytophan available in the body. Add more complex carbohydrates (lower protein) along with carbohydrate-digesting enzymes.

- Consider tryptophan or 5-HTP supplements. If you are taking other medications of any type, check with your doctor first.

- Consider an SSRI medication if other avenues do not work. If 5-HTP causes a change but you have trouble getting consistent results, this may indicate an SSRI trial may be helpful.

- If you do not exercise, begin some sort of exercise program. Something like walking 30 minutes a few times a week may make a noticeable difference.

Situation 11. Interactions between medications, supplements, and enzymes

In general, enzymes do not interact directly with supplements or medications because the other products are not appropriate targets (substrates) for them. However, there might be some indirect actions.

1. Since enzymes can enhance the absorption and use of any food, supplements, or medications, your body might actually be getting a slightly larger dose of the supplement or medicine consumed. Often you can reduce the amount of the supplement or medicine to get the same results as before.

2. Enzymes may eliminate the reason you need the supplement or medication. For example, if the supplement or medication is given to help sleep or anxiety problems, the enzymes may end the sleep or anxiety problems, and so the other product is no longer needed.

3. Some time-released medications use cellulose in them to impart the time-release function - a functional use of cellulose. If cellulose is used as a functional part of the time-release product, you need to avoid enzyme products containing the enzyme cellulase. Cellulase enzymes may breakdown the time-release medication right away disrupting how the medication works. You can ask your pharmacist if your time-release medication contains cellulose as a functional part of the medication. Pancreatic enzymes do not contain cellulase. Lypo (*Enzymedica*) can serve as a broad-spectrum enzyme product that also does not contain cellulase. You may need to take a couple of enzyme products without cellulase to get the mix of enzymes you want. An example is taking Lypo plus GlutenEase or Peptizyde along with time-release seizure medication.

   Note: Some products use a blend called CereCalase(TM). CereCalase contains cellulase. If you are unsure about an exact enzyme name or blend, wait until you check with the manufacturer on the types of enzymes the product contains before using it.

4. If you are taking blood thinning medications, consult your health practitioner before starting strong proteases or nattokinase products.

more . . .

Should I start enzymes first or supplements/medications?

If you are already taking a supplement or medication, you do not need to stop if you want to add in enzymes. However, if you have started neither enzymes nor the other items, start the enzymes first. After you are adjusted to enzymes, add in the other supplements or medications one at a time. Enzymes can increase absorption and utilization of everything you put in your mouth (supplements, medications, and foods including diet foods). Enzymes may improve the effectiveness of the supplements or medications. If you start enzymes first, you will be better able to determine if the supplement or medication is helping and what dose you need. If you start the supplement or medication first, the body may not be absorbing and using it well and its benefits may not be evident.

Supplements or medications over time

You may find that supplements or medications are not needed over time after starting enzymes. It is reasonable to eventually need less enzymes over time as well. As the gut heals and intestinal function improves, absorption improves too. The nutrient deficiencies that supplements aimed to correct are now being addressed by nutrition from food. Some supplements may even begin to cause problems after several months taking enzymes because they are now contributing to an excess amount of a particular nutrient. Vitamin B6 given at very high doses is a particular supplement that tends to cause problems after several months with enzymes. The excessively high doses of B6 become unnecessary. You can reduce the B6 to a more typical level, or drop it altogether.

Situation 12. Head-banging, head sensitivity

Related Symptoms
1. Bangs head repetitively, often with force on hard surfaces.
2. Dislikes clothing pulled over head.
3. Dislikes hair and face washing.
4. Dislikes kisses, hugs, or affection around the head area.
5. May be hypersensitive to light, sounds, visual displays, color.
6. May act as though they have hearing problems.
7. May have oral sensory issues, or chew excessively (the chewies).
8. May have screaming fits which start without any apparent reason, and nothing seems to calm the person or stop the fits.

When I hear of head-banging, I think pain. Pain in the head, such as with a migraine, severe headache, toothache, etc., can cause a multitude of sensory problems all associated with a hypersensitive head zone.

Think of an adult who has a migraine. Typical reactions are to stay in a dark quiet room, nausea or vomiting, and irritability. The last thing a person with a migraine wants to do is have lots of conversation, go shopping at the mall, or socialize. When adults verbalize they have a serious headache or migraine, or just had lots of work done to them at the dentist, people around them know to make allowances for the suffering person.

Children are unable to communicate their head pain in the same way. A toddler is not going to say, "Mommy, I have a migraine with intense throbbing and visual disturbances!" A child will only know he or she is in intense pain, act out, withdraw from socializing, and may start banging their head to get some relief from the pain.

A child will not want to play with others or communicate just as an adult does not in a similar situation. A child will not be doing well in other therapies, may appear to have attention problems, and will not be participating in school. This is just like an adult not being very productive at work when they have head pain.

Often head pain interrupts good sleep. My neurologist explained to me that during proper sleep, the body produces pain regulating compounds that affect how the body interprets/processes/perceives

more . . .

pain, or process sensory input signals. Fixing the sleep often corrects the impaired pain interpretation signaling, which in turn, helps you get better sleep. *see page 255*

What to do suggestions

- Epsom salts or melatonin - addressing sleep problems may help with pain management and sensory issues. Fixing the sleep may help many other sensory issues and pain interpretation problems go away. *see Sleep problems, page 255*

- Medications for head pain, such as amitryptiline which is used for sleep disorders and pain, may offer temporary relief and improve quality of life while you pursue locating an underlying cause. See a specialist in childhood migraines or head pain.

- Enzymes and probiotics may help resolve gut and food intolerances triggering the head pain. Artificial additives often trigger pain.

- Magnesium - may help with pain.

- Essential fatty acids.

- Treating a yeast, bacteria, or viral problem may relieve the source of the distress.

- Sensory management - small adjustments can go a long way. Wear soft clothing that does not go over the head, and pants that are loose and roomy (climber and cargo pants are roomy and come in several colors and textures - L.L. Bean or sporting goods stores carry these). Limit sensory input; do not push the person to deal with more than he can. Rougher textured clothing or softer textured clothing may be helpful depending on the individual sensitivities.

- Special sensory therapy may help - auditory processing therapy, checking vision.

- Correct any encopresis or bowel impaction. *see pages 236-240*

Situation 13. Child chews his clothes, the furniture, wallpaper, the cat's tail, and just about anything in sight - The Chewies

Related Symptoms

1. A child may chronically chew his clothes to shreds. Usually this is the shirt collar or sleeves that look 'eaten' with saliva soaked extensively into the shirt.
2. May also have what looks like an anxiety problem.
3. May also 'eat everything in site'; act as if he is constantly hungry; may prefer hard, crunchy foods.
4. Teeth grinding; bruxism.

The child may not even realize he is doing this. If you ask him why he is gnawing on some non-food item in his mouth, he may be as surprised as anyone he is doing it.

This chewing problem may be resolved in several ways. The quickest and often most inexpensive is to try minerals - first magnesium and if that does not work, try zinc. Calcium has solved the problem in a few cases.

If the person has head pain, migraines, or some other chronic discomfort, he may be chewing to try to counter this pain. This is similar to when you hurt a part of your body, you instantly grab it with your hands and start applying pressure to numb out the pain. If the pain is in the head, crunching hard foods or ice, chewing on objects, or head-banging may be a method for trying to get some relief from the pain.

If the person acts constantly hungry, this may be a need to chew on something and not actual hunger.

Personal experience:

I personally suffered chronic migraines for several decades before being prescribed amitryptiline which helped immensely. The idea was to correct the sleep and pain sensory interpretation system. My son was a chronic head-banger and this medication helped him greatly as well. He stopped banging his head at night, his sleep improved, and his debilitating sensory sensitivities drop by about 50% in the first week.

more . . .

In addition, my neurologist prescribed magnesium, and told me to look for possible sensory 'triggers.' One of our migraine triggers was dairy. This problem was eliminated by using enzymes for dairy. The addition of extra proteases between meals helped as well (around nine capsules or more a day between meals). The combination of medication, magnesium, enzymes and sensory management made the head-banging, chewies, and migraines a thing of the past.

What to do suggestions

- Magnesium supplement - magnesium may relieve the chewies directly. It may also assist indirectly with the chewies by relaxing the muscles which relieves what appears to be an anxiety driven need to chew. see Magnesium, page 264

- If magnesium does not correct this, try zinc. see Zinc deficiency, page 266

- If minerals are not the solution, look into sensory therapy with an appropriate occupational therapist. It could be an oral motor or sensory problem. Sensory therapy for chewing objects and exercises are available.

- Some people report a yeast, bacteria, or viral problem can cause the chewies. You can investigate further if you have reason to suspect one of these issues.

Situation 14. Magnesium deficiency

Related Symptoms
1. Muscle tension, restless leg, pains, the 'chewies.'
2. May appear to have anxiety problems or obsessive behaviors.
3. Sleeping problems.
4. Migraines or chronic pain.
5. Prone to constipation problems.

Magnesium deficiency is very common in the general population and particularly prevalent in children with behavior problems, neurological, and autoimmune conditions.

Several research studies confirm that a therapeutic use of magnesium has proven effective for migraines, negative hyperactivity, autism conditions, anxiety, and autoimmune problems.

One function of magnesium is to help balance out calcium for proper muscle movement. Calcium helps muscles to contract while magnesium helps muscles to relax. Calcium is added to several food products whereas magnesium is often overlooked. Calcium is stored in the body whereas magnesium is water-soluble and washes out. So it is easy to become deficient in magnesium whereas calcium can accumulate in the body. This can lead to tense muscles because the magnesium is not present to balance the muscles out.

What appears as 'anxiety' or 'anxiety disorder' may actually be a person with too little magnesium to sufficiently relax their muscles. Their disposition appears tense because their muscles are physically taut. When the person adds a therapeutic amount of magnesium, the muscles physically relax and the previous anxiety appears to go away. Restless leg, muscle spasms, involuntary twitching movements, shooting pains as well as some obsessive repetitive behaviors might be resolved by trying inexpensive magnesium therapy.

This balance of muscle movement is needed in the gut as well. Lack of magnesium can lead to constipation problems. Adding sufficient magnesium for good bowel regularity is a good way to determine your personal dosage level.

more . . .

A commonly overlooked situation that can drive a magnesium deficiency or make it worse is when a person removes dairy or whole grains from their diet. When dairy is removed, the person is usually aware of the need for calcium and will start supplementing calcium. However, without additional magnesium to balance out the calcium, this increased calcium can lead to more magnesium deficiency. When whole grains are eliminated, a major source of magnesium may be lost.

What to do suggestions

- Magnesium supplements - a well-absorbed form, not oxide; the therapeutic dose is 1,000 mg per day. Start the magnesium at 100 mg and increase by 100 mg at a time until you get regular loose stools. Then back down a bit on the dose. This is your personal threshold for magnesium.

Magnesium supplements come in many forms and potencies (tablets, powders, liquids, etc). Natural Calm is a highly absorbable liquid available in several flavors. Tablets and capsules come in a wide range of sizes. Magnesium malate may have an extra benefit of assisting in the removal of excess heavy metals such as aluminum. Magnesium glycinate is thought to help with gut healing. Magnesium chelate is thought to have enhanced absorption. Most any form can work, however, avoid magnesium oxide because it is poorly absorbed. The main factor is to find a well-absorbed source of magnesium that works for your situation.

- Epsom salts - either as a bath, lotion, or skin wash. The magnesium is absorbed through the skin. While this can be quite helpful, the dose may not be nearly high enough for a therapeutic use. You can take Epsom salts and magnesium supplements together. Epsom salts at bedtime can help the muscles relax sufficiently for better sleep.

Situation 15. Zinc deficiency

Related Symptoms
1. May have 'the chewies.' *see page 262*
2. Constantly getting sick with lots of various illnesses.
3. Leaky gut, many food intolerances or chemical sensitivities.
4. White spots on fingernails.
5. Wounds slow to heal.
6. High copper levels or excess levels of other heavy metals.

Zinc is needed to support the immune system, fight illnesses, and maintain intestinal integrity. Substantial research shows supplementing zinc assists in healing intestinal tissue. Zinc is an essential co-factor in many enzyme reactions and also functions as an antioxidant. One of these zinc compounds functions to grab and remove heavy metals attempting to enter our bodies. The metal binder is known as metallothionein and requires seven zinc atoms. It is located in the gut at the base of the villi, among other locations.

Zinc as well as magnesium is often woefully deficient in many children with behavioral problems, and most neurological and autoimmune conditions.

What to do suggestions

• Zinc supplements - add in slowly. Increasing the zinc dose too rapidly can lead to copper being displaced quicker than the body can process it out. This can cause adverse reactions.

With zinc, the RDA range is 2 to 15 mg a day with 50 mg per day being the upper limit for children and 100 mg for adults (before toxicity problems can occur). Start with the RDA amount of zinc and increase by 3 to 5 mg at a time to around 30 to 40 mg. If you are interested in dosing above the RDA, please check with your health practitioner for your situation.

Situation 16. Problems with eyes or eye contact

Related Symptoms
1. Hand-flapping in area of peripheral vision.
2. Eye twitching, problems focusing with eyes.
3. May show problems with depth perception.
4. May appear to have problems with hearing, or deafness even if hearing tests come back as okay.
5. May have sensory issues around their head - doesn't like shirts over the head, washing face, washing hair, kisses on face.

Visual problems may be due to several causes. Sometimes a supplement can help. Other times, it is not dietary or nutrition related. Non-dietary avenues to pursue would be to do a thorough eye check, or look into a special vision aid called Irlen lenses. When examining vision, most people think to check the physical functioning of the eyes. However, also check neurological causes of problems with visual sensory processing.

What to do suggestions

Supplements that tend to help eye issues are:
- essential fatty acids (EFA, DHA, omega 3)
- cod liver oil
- vitamin A

- Check for issues related to head pain.
  see Head-banging, page 260

- Check for issues related to auditory processing or hearing.

- Check for issues related to motor coordination or balance.

Situation 17. Problems with language or speech

Related Symptoms
1. Problems forming words or sentences.
2. Problems using words appropriately (echolalia, video talk).
3. May appear to have problems with hearing, deafness even if hearing tests come back as okay.
4. May have sensory issues around their head.

Below are some supplement suggestions which tend to work for language problems. With essential fatty acids, the brand quality can make a big difference. Nordic Naturals and Barleans are two high quality brands specializing in oils and having a large selection of products. The type of fatty acid can make a big difference as well. If one type of oil or brand does not give good results, try at least one other. Also, try giving lipase enzymes with the oils to enhance their absorption.

DMG and TMG focus on improving methylation. DMG has two methyl groups and TMG has three. Sometimes DMG will work when TMG does not, and vice versa.

A study with Carn-Aware demonstrated how language improved in individuals with autism. A few participants also showed improvement in seizures. (Chez, Buchanan, and Aimonovitch 2002).

What to do suggestions

Supplements that tend to help language besides digestive enzymes are:
- essential fatty acids (EFA, DHA, omega 3)
- carnosine plus zinc (such as Carn-Aware)
- DMG or TMG

- Check for issues related to head pain.
  see Head-banging, page 260

Situation 18. Is malabsorption the same as leaky gut?

Related Symptoms

1. Food sensitivities or allergy tests coming back with a huge number of sensitivities.
2. Adverse reactions to 'everything.'
3. Yeast, bacteria, chronic illness; constant vague health problems, person just cannot seem to get well.

Although you can have both conditions, and they are related, they are technically different. Leaky gut can be caused by a variety of things and can very often lead to malabsorption. Leaky gut is the state where the protective gut lining loses its integrity. It is less capable of properly screening out those elements that should be blocked, and allowing in only the proper elements. Items that should be screened out 'leak' through into the body.

Malabsorption means 'bad absorption of some type for some reason.' It does not indicate the cause. It simply means at least some nutrients are not being absorbed properly. Leaky gut may be involved, but you can also have malabsorption without leaky gut. If you have a pancreatic problem, poor stomach acid, various diseases, or other causes, you might have an intact gut lining but for some other reason, some nutrients are not being absorbed properly. This might be many nutrients or only a few in particular.

What is nice about digestive enzymes is they can help both a leaky gut and malabsorption at the same time.

What to do suggestions

- Probiotics, enzymes.

- Zinc.

- Essential fatty acids.

- Reduce or eliminate artificial additives, refined and highly processed foods.

- Avoid hydrogenated fats.

Situation 19. Thirst/loose stools/constipation/irregular bowels when starting enzymes

Related Symptoms
1. Foul stench to stools.
2. Stools containing compounds of various colors, textures, or consistencies, including mucus.

Enzymes help the body metabolize more food and liquid. You may find you need to drink more liquid now. A few people see temporary increased wetting or urination. Looser stools may also occur in the first few days and may last up to two weeks. This is not the same as diarrhea, just looser stools. Also, as any debris gets removed from the intestines, you may have a few days where stools have assorted colors, textures, and substances in them. This can include brightly colored pieces, stringy substances, mucus, dark specks, frothy stools, or any number of assorted types of material with interesting properties. Do not be alarmed as this is a common part of intestinal 'house-cleaning.'

If the interesting stools do not stabilize by the second to third week (allow a bit longer with yeast overgrowth), reduce the enzymes, or stop them completely, and seek assistance. Usually other symptoms or behaviors are also present to let you know if this is part of normal adjustments effects or not. Also, check Chapter 16, Studying Stools, for the possible meaning of specific stool conditions.

What to do suggestions

- Allow a few weeks for your body to adjust to taking enzymes and get through the 'house-cleaning' phase. If constipation or loose stools persist past this, reduce the dose of enzymes and see if that helps.

- Drink eight to ten glasses of water a day. Constipation may occur if not enough liquid is passing through your system. Liquid is needed to help soften stools and flow digested contents through the intestinal tract.

more . . .

• With stool stench, consider doing some sort of antibiotic to treat for harmful bacteria. Ten days of Source Naturals colloidal silver worked very well for my family. Others have had similar success with this method especially with persistent bacteria problems. Colloidal silver is a metal, if this is a concern, although people undertaking detoxification programs have relayed colloidal silver has not been a problem when they used it short-term for bacteria problems. Be sure to research the brand you are considering and see if it is right for your situation. Other antibiotics are available over-the-counter as well as by prescription.

• With perceived constipation, try to determine if it is true constipation or just less waste coming out. Enzymes, particularly the fiber digesting enzymes, break down more food which is used by your body. This means there would be less total matter coming out. A good bowel elimination pattern is one to two stools each one to two days.

• If true constipation persists after starting enzymes, consider adding magnesium. Magnesium deficiency can contribute to constipation. Since many people are magnesium deficient, this deficiency may not become apparent until some basic digestive problems are improved, such as what can happen when starting enzymes. See Magnesium, page 264, in this book, and the magnesium chapter in *Enzymes for Autism/ Digestive Health*.

• Some medications cause constipation or diarrhea as a side-effect. Check any medications to see if this is a factor. Since enzymes improve absorption of many substances, more medication may be getting absorbed and contributing to constipation or diarrhea. Ask your doctor about reducing the dose of medication.

Situation 20. Chronic constipation or encopresis without enzymes or before starting enzymes

Related Symptoms

1. Constipation to the extreme; more than a couple months duration.
2. Bowel movements are accompanied by a horrendous stench. So foul you want to run out of the house. Stench indicates bacteria.
3. Bowel movement, when it does occur, produces a mass so large it frequently clogs up the toilet, or simply cannot pass down. Mass tends to be very clay-like and dense. Usually very painful for person.

This situation of constipation out of control, or encopresis, is more common than one might think. It often appears in young children but can be frequent in adults too. Unless treated, it rarely gets better on its own. The remedy is not expensive or hard, but does require persistance.

What to do suggestions

- Add a laxative of some sort at a rate high enough to keep stool moving out regularly. I prefer magnesium as it helps with other deficiency symptoms and is safe. If there is serious impaction, you may prefer to do an initial colon cleanse or impaction removal process.

- It is critical for the person to follow a 'bathroom schedule.' About 10 minutes after eating a meal, the person needs to 'try' on the toilet for about 10 minutes. It is not important whether anything comes out, but it is important to keep this schedule of 'trying.' This process helps to retrain the bowel muscles and allow the colon to shrink back into the proper shape and function. This process is needed for a minimum of six months. Giving up on the bathroom schedule too early is the main reason for this method failing and the problem returning. see Encopresis, page 236

- Include appropriate amounts of fiber in the diet along with the needed water to keep stool soft and moving.

Situation 21. Throwing up right after taking enzymes

Related Symptoms
1. Chronic acid stomach or nausea.
2. Candida yeast or bacteria problems.
3. Fungus on fingernails or toenails.
4. Problems digesting carbohydrates.

This is a rare occurrance but it has been reported. An explanation for this was offered by a fellow who worked many years in the supplement industry and several years working with a specialist in *Candida* yeast problems. He commented that if there is yeast or bacteria in the stomach or throat area, and you take something that helps kill these pathogens, such as enzymes, probiotics, or certain anti-pathogen herbs, it can cause some throwing up in the beginning. The anti-pathogen supplements cause some die-off and your body is trying to expel the crud as quickly as possible. If the harmful microbes are located in the lower intestines and bowel, you may experience diarrhea or some very interesting looking stools for a few days. If the pathogens are located in the upper GI tract, the residue may come out topside.

What to do suggestions

- Treat the problem as a die-off reaction and continue any die-off control measures you may be following (such as Epsom salts or antioxidants).

- If you are not currently treating for harmful yeast, bacteria, or parasites, look into the possibility that one of these is a problem. If so, implement an appropriate pathogen control program.

- Reduce the dose of the enzymes, probiotics, or herbs so the reaction can proceed at a more tolerable rate. You may need to give only a very little bit at a time. You may need to start with as little as 1/8 to 1/16 of a typical dose.

Situation 22. Reflux or GERD

Related Symptoms
1. Chronic acid stomach.
2. Stomach or gut tightening or cramping after eating.

My younger son had chronic reflux for about seven years until he started enzymes regularly. It did not go away overnight, but the reflux was much less by the second month. In the third month, it was even less. By the fourth month, it had pretty much stopped and did not come back anymore. That was three and a half years ago. Several older adults have told me their reflux ended following a similar pattern with enzymes.

You might want to consider a 'gentler' low-protease enzyme product initially. Something like Lacto or V-Gest (*Enzymedica*). Then, after one bottle of that, switch to something with more proteases like Digest Gold (*Enzymedica*), Elite-Zyme Ultra (*Thropp's*), Vital-zymes Complete (*Klaire Labs*) or something similar. Starting with something gentler, particularly in the case of children, initially tends to be better tolerated until a little more healing takes place. With reflux, the main thing seems to be just sticking with the enzymes regularly for a few months.

What to do suggestions

- Take a good broad-spectrum digestive enzyme product for two to three months. You may notice a difference right away, although the problem tends to become gradually less intense and less frequent as you continue enzymes regularly with all meals (and snacks if possible). *see The Great Low-n-Slow Method, Chapter 6*

- If you are taking something for immediate relief, such as antacid or a prescription medication, continue taking that while the enzymes work on healing. There are some enzymes designed for short-term immediate relief of acid stomach.

- For temporary quick relief, try taking 1/8 teaspoon of kitchen cabinet baking soda to neutralize excess acid.

Situation 23. Pain or stomach ache occurs when you start enzymes. What to do with gastritis

Related Symptoms
1. Rarely, may be reflux, vomiting, or nausea.
2. Pain may be an acute period stinging, or general ache.
3. Concern enzymes are digesting internal tissue away.

Sometimes after starting a strong protease enzyme product, the person may have a stomach ache or pain. Although proteases such as bromelain and papain have been used extensively to heal gastric ulcers, proteases in particular may initially irritate the gut a little. For why this may happen, see pages 98 to100. *see The Great Low-n-Slow Method*

What to do suggestions

- If enzymes were taken on an empty stomach when the discomfort occurred, try taking the enzymes with food for a few days. Sometimes taking them with meals for the first week or two helps during the adjustment period even with enzymes intended to be taken between meals.

- Stop the enzymes completely for four to five days. Then start again at a lower dose and work up gradually to the full dose. This allows the clean but raw and exposed tissue time to heal up a bit and be less sensitive.

- If re-starting the initial enzyme product still causes pain, park the enzymes your are using on a shelf. Switch to a product low in proteases (V-Gest or Lacto tend to work the very best). After finishing 10 days of V-Gest or Lacto, or one bottle's worth, continue with the previous enzyme product again. This resolves the pain in the vast majority of cases.

- Consider a short trial of some gut soothing products, such as Acid-Soothe enzymes, aloe vera products, slippery elm and other herbs, you may want to consider.

- For temporary quick relief of acid stomach, try taking 1/8 teaspoon of baking soda to neutralize excess acid.

Situation 24. Concern about how protease enzymes distinguish among proteins in the body

Some people wonder how protease enzymes distinguish among proteins? The thinking is if our insides consist of proteins, will protease enzyme supplements start digesting our own bodies away? The answer is no, this does not happen. Enzymes are very very specific. There may be an assumption that all proteases work on all proteins no matter what. This is the opposite of what actually happens. There are thousands of very different proteins and even more unique proteases. Only certain proteases work on certain types of proteins, and only under certain conditions. The chemical and physical structure of both the enzyme and the target as well as the environment has to be exactly right in order for the enzyme to work at all. Enzymes are not interchangeable. Much like an electrician, a carpenter, and a mason all work to build a house, their jobs and skills are not interchangeable.

There are checks and balances throughout the body regulating all enzymes, not just proteases and not just in the digestive tract. This is a reason enzymes are considered incredibly safe. They do not wander around the body doing who knows what as other supplements or medications can. This also contributes to the very few true side-effects seen with enzymes.

On the very practical side, consider this: If any protease could digest our own healthy tissue, our forefathers would have eaten once. After that initial bite, our own proteases produced by the pancreas would have kicked into action, digested the food, and then proceeded to digest all other body parts. We would already have digested away long ago. But that does not happen. Even people with very serious gut problems have pancreatic proteases being churned out daily if not hourly, and yet they do not digest away.

When food is cooked, it is changed chemically and structurally. With proteins, the three-dimensional structure is damaged. The protein looses its configuration and sort of unravels. Make a tight fist and think of this as a protein. In this form, digestive enzymes cannot reach the inside palm of your hand to break it down. Now, relax the fist and spread out your fingers. This is similar to what happens when food, or

more . . .

proteins, are cooked and the protein becomes damaged. Now enzymes can access the palm of your hand directly.

This is also true even if you have very injured intestinal tissue. In the situation with exposed healthy tissue, the healthy proteins are tender because of exposed nerves. But the proteins still retains its structure so the enzymes cannot access the appropriate bonds and break the protein down. If the tissue is dead, damaged, or infected, it looses the protective configuration and thus the protease enzymes can help break down the debris and clean out the gunk.

Situation 25. Someone told me digestive enzyme supplements do not work because they are destroyed by the stomach acid

This is a common point of confusion. Many health professionals learned about pancreatic enzymes in their training. If you start talking about 'enzymes' they may understandably assume you mean pancreatic ones. Then, they may tell you since the enzymes you are taking are not enterically coated, they are destroyed in the stomach and worthless. This is true for pancreatic enzymes, which are usually enterically coated to protect them, but it is not true for plant or microbial-derived enzymes. So it depends entirely on the type of enzyme used and how it is manufactured. There have been many advances in enzyme therapy in the past decade alone. Advances some people may not be aware of.

Pancreatic enzymes are a type of digestive enzyme derived from animals. There are FDA approved prescription pancreatic enzymes as well as pancreatic products sold over-the-counter. However, most digestive enzyme products sold over-the-counter are plant and microbial-derived. These are not destroyed in the stomach and are more stable at a wide range of pH and temperature. These enzymes can give stunning improvements in digestion, pathogen control, and chronic illnesses. Another difference between pancreatic and microbial-derived enzymes is pancreatic enzymes come in a set ratio of amylases, proteases, and lipases, whereas microbial enzymes can be customized for various uses.

Situation 26. Do improvements with enzymes wear off over time?

Often a person wonders if the positive improvements seen with enzymes in the beginning will last. The question of 'do enzymes wear off' was heavily monitored in the first year of the enzymes and autism discussion group. But since May 2001 and thousands of families, this has never been reported. There are no reports of this in any of the clinical literature either. There was also a concern that a person may become 'intolerant' of enzymes over time as they do to many foods. This also has never been reported.

What we see after thousands of cases and over five years experience is if an enzyme product is not going to work, or has limited benefits, this is apparent from the beginning. There has been no record of abrupt regression several months later as does happen at times if you follow a GFCF diet and then quit the diet without enzymes. If enzymes do work from the beginning, the improvements remain over time, or continue to improve more over time.

Enzymes can help pro-actively heal tissue. So what you may see is that the longer you use enzymes, the less enzymes you need for the same level of improvement. This may be due to gut healing. As the gut heals, your own enzymes can be restored so you do not need supplemental ones as much.

Occasionally, improvements with enzymes seem to 'disappear' after several months. In every case reported, this eventually was traced to another cause and not the enzymes. Causes included a vacation trip, new therapy, a cold or virus going around, new supplement or medication, starting school, exposure to new food or chemical, or some other source. Once the other source was dealt with, the improvements seen with enzymes return.

If you are taking high doses of another supplement or medication, that supplement or medicine may not be needed now after being on enzymes. With gut healing and improved absorption, the dose you were taking before may now be too high and so causing problems. This often happens particularly with high doses of B6. You can try removing or reducing the dose and see if that helps.

Situation 27. Fungal-derived enzymes and *Aspergillus* sensitivity or mold allergy

Related Symptoms
1. Food sensitivities or allergy tests coming back with a huge number of sensitivities.
2. *Candida* overgrowth.

Most allergies are defense reactions to some type of protein (or part of a protein). Any protein in nature can potentially be an allergen. Enzymes are proteins that do work. So potentially, any enzyme could be an allergen for any individual just like any other protein. However, digestive enzymes occur in our bodies and in our food all the time throughout our lives, they are far less likely to be an allergen than most proteins.

Enzymes are extensively purified so there is no or negligible trace of contamination of any part of the source in the final product. Most people with mold or yeast allergies do not have any problem with fungal-derived enzymes. However, a few people do have reactions. It is completely understandable if this is something you do not wish to risk. Only you can determine if it is right for your situation. If you decide against using enzymes from fungal sources, you still have the option of pancreatic enzymes, plant-derived enzymes (bromelain, papain, actinidin), or bacterial-derived enzymes.

More people having a specific sensitivity to *Aspergillus* have told me they do have problems with enzymes derived from this organism. With *Aspergillus* sensitivity, consider enzymes from another source, such as pancreatic, plant, or bacterial-derived enzymes.

Sometimes a person who is sensitive to *Aspergillus* or mold is also reactive to 'everything' because of a poor immune system, leaky gut, or other condition which leads to an overworked immune system. Taking enzymes helps overall health. This improvement reduces the total load on the immune system so it can 'react' appropriately. This adjustment then reduces or eliminates the *Aspergillus* or mold sensitivity. In these situations, taking fungal-derived digestive enzymes helps reduce the mold sensitivity rather than cause an adverse reaction.

Situation 28. Picking an enzyme product

The following process will help you narrow down which products to consider. Writing your answers down on paper may help greatly.

Part 1. Identify what problem you want to address with enzymes.
Select an enzyme product based on what results you want to achieve. Digestion of specific foods? Inflammation? Viral, bacteria, or yeast control? Enzyme products can be mixed and matched, so you do not have to buy everything from one company or get everything from one product.

Part 2. Identify what types of enzymes will work on the problem you want to address.
For example, if you struggle with yeast, look at the yeast program and the enzymes designed for yeast control. If it is fat digestion, consider a broad-spectrum product high in lipases, or a general broad-spectrum product plus a separate product specifically for fat digestion.

Part 3. Identify what products contain the types of enzymes you need to work on the problem you want to address.
After you find one or more appropriate products, further narrow down the choices by considering the following:

a. See if the products contain any fillers or other added ingredients that you cannot tolerate. Things like rice bran, MCT oil, herbs, fruit-derived enzymes, or other supplemented nutrients included in the formulation may make a product off-limits for you.

b. Check with other sources with a situation close to yours and see how the product has performed for actual users.

c. Look closely at the amount of activity of the enzymes and how many capsules consititute a 'serving' so you will have a good idea of how many enzymes you will be actually be taking.

more . . .

d. Once you have one or more possible choices, try one bottle of a product. You are usually able to tell if it is helping with one bottle's worth. If you had a second close choice, try one bottle of that product next, and so on. Then go with whichever product worked the best for your situation. Allow time for adjustments and refining your program as you go. Again, writing things down and keeping a log or journal can help you see patterns you may not otherwise detect.

Note: See the www.enzymestuff.com site for additional information. Also, joining the enzymes discussion group connects you to many other families using enzymes for their situations.
http://group.yahoo.com/group/enzymesandautism

Situation 29. What should I try first? Best bets when starting

Related Symptoms
1. Totally confused over what to do. All the supplements and diets sound 'essential.'
2. Have limited funds, time, and energy.
3. Ready to scream wildly and bang head on the floor for hours.

Digestive enzymes are an excellent first step measure. They can eliminate the need for many food removals while dealing with many digestive problems across the board. Enzymes can alleviate the need for many supplements and help you get the most value from the ones you do take. Besides digestive enzymes, there are some other best bet measures. The following are derived from years of research and experience. These tend to cover the most issues for the most people - the most bang for your buck (in terms of health and healing). These are inexpensive, safe measures you can do right away that go a long way toward helping overall health. After doing these, see what is left over and focus on those areas. These focus only on biological/nutritional avenues and can be done in conjunction with other measures (such as educational therapy, medications, physical therapy, pain management, and so on).

What to do suggestions

- Digestive enzymes.

- Probiotics - either as a supplement on in a whole-food source.

- Epsom salts - cheap and easy; more directions and discussion in *Enzymes for Autism/Digestive Health*, and at www.enzymestuff.com/epsomsalts.htm.

- Magnesium - a soluble form, see page 264.

- Zinc - see page 266.

- Essential fatty acids - omega-3s, fish oils, cod liver oil, etc.; avoid hydrogenated fats.

- Sleep - see page 255.

- Hypoglycemia - see page 245.

References

Alles, M.S., Hautvast, J.G.A., Nagengast, F.M., Hartemink, R., Van Laere, K.M., and Jansen, J.B. 1996. 'Fate of fructo-oligosaccharides in the human intestine.' *British Journal of Nutrition* 76:211-21.

Andrews, G.K. 2000. 'Regulation of metallothionein gene expression by oxidative stress and metal ions.' *Biochemical Pharmacology* 59:95-104.

Banchini, G., Scaricabarozzi, I., Montecorboli, U., Ceccarelli, A., Chiesa, F., Ditri, L., Mazzer, G., Moroni, R., Viola, M., Roggia, F., *et al.* 1993. 'Double-blind study of nimesulide in divers with inflammatory disorders of the ear, nose and throat.' *Drugs* 46(Suppl 1):100-2.

Baranyi, M., Thomas, U., and Pellegrini, A. 2003. 'Antibacterial activity of casein-derived peptides isolated from rabbit (*Oryctolagus cuniculus*) milk.' *Journal of Dairy Research* May 70(2):189-97.

Bearcroft, C.P., Perrett, D., and Farthing, M.J.G. 1998. 'Postprandial plasma 5-hydroxytryptamine in diarrhea predominant irritable bowel syndrome: a pilot study.' *Gut* 42:42-46.

Bleichner, G., Blehaut, H., Mentec, H., and Moyse, D. 1997. '*Saccharomyces boulardii* prevents diarrhea in critically ill tube-fed patients. A multicenter, randomized, double-blind placebo-controlled trial.' *Intensive Care Medicine* 23:517–23.

Booth, S.L., and Centurelli, M.A. 1999. 'Vitamin K: a practical guide to the dietary management of patients on warfarin.' *Nutrition Review* 57(9 Pt 1):288-296.

Bracale, G. and Selvetella, L. 1996. 'Clinical study of the efficacy of and tolerance to seaprose S in inflammatory venous disease. Controlled study versus serratio-peptidase.' *Minerva Cardioangiologica* October 44(10):515-24.

Braga, P.C., Piatti, G., Grasselli, G., Casali, W., Beghi, G., and Allegra, L. 1992. 'The influence of seaprose on erythromycin penetration into bronchial mucus in bronchopulmonary infections.' *Drugs Under Experimental and Clinical Research* 18(3):105-11.

Brody, T. 1999. *Nutritional Biochemistry* 2nd edition. San Diego, California. Academic Press.

Byun, T., Kofod, L., and Blinkovsky, A. 2001. 'Synergistic action of an X-prolyl dipeptidyl aminopeptidase and a non-specific aminopeptidase in a protein hydrolysis.' *Journal of Agriculture and Food Chemistry* 49(4):2061-2063.

Carlson, M.S., Hill, G.M., and Link, J.E. 1999. 'Early- and traditionally weaned nursery pigs benefit from phase-feeding pharmacological concentrations of zinc oxide: effect on metallothionein and mineral concentrations.' *Journal of Animal Science* May 77(5):1199-207.

Carlson, M.S., Hoover, S.L., Hill, G.M., Link, J.E., and Turk, J.R. 1998. 'Effect of pharmacological zinc on intestinal metallothionein concentration and morphology in the nursery pig.' *Journal of Animal Science* 76(Suppl 1):57 Abstr.

Case, C.L., and Carlson, M.S. 2002. 'Effect of feeding organic and inorganic sources of additional zinc on growth performance and zinc balance in nursery pigs.' *Journal of Animal Science* 80:1917-1924.

Castagliuolo, I., Reigler, M.F., Valenick, L., LaMont, J.T., and Pothoulakis, C. 1999. '*Saccharomyces boulardii* protease inhibits the effects of *Clostridium difficile* toxins A and B in human colonic mucosa.' *Infection and Immunity* January 67(1):302-7.

Castell, J.V., Friedrich, G., Kuhn, C.S., and Poppe, G.E. 1997. 'Intestinal absorption of undegraded proteins in men: presence of bromelain in plasma after oral intake.' Unidad de Hepatologia Experimental, Hospital Universitario La Fe, Valencia, Spain. *American Journal of Physiology* July 273(1 Pt 1):G139-46.

Chez, M.G., Buchanan, C.P., Aimonovitch, M.C., Becker, M., Schaefer, K., Black, C., and Komen, J. 2002. 'Double-blind, placebo-controlled study of L-carnosine supplementation in children with autistic spectrum disorders.' *Journal of Child Neurology* November 17(11):833-7.

Cousins, R. J. 1985. 'Absorption, transport and hepatic metabolism of copper and zinc: special reference to metallothionein and ceruloplasmin.' *Physiological Reviews* 65:238-309.

Davis, S.R., and Cousins, R.J. 2000. 'Metallothionein Expression in Animals: A Physiological Perspective on Function.' *Journal of Nutrition* 130:1085-1088.

Danielson, K.G., Ohi, S., and Huang, P.C. 1982. 'Immunochemical detection of metallothionein in specific epithelial cells of rat organs.' *Proceedings of the National Academy of Science USA* April 79(7):2301–2304.

Desser, L., Holomanova, D., Zavadova, E., Pavelka, K., Mohr, T., and Herbacek, I. 2001. 'Oral therapy with proteolytic enzymes decreases excessive TGF-beta levels in human blood.' Institute of Cancer Research, University of Vienna, Austria. *Cancer Chemotherapy and Pharmacology* July 47(Suppl):S10-5.

Desser, L., and Rehberger, A. 1990. 'Induction of tumor necrosis factor in human peripheral-blood mononuclear cells by proteolytic enzymes.' *Oncology* 47(6):475-7.

Dial, E.J., Hall, L.R., Serna, H., Romero, J.J., Fox, J.G., and Lichtenberger, L. 1998. 'Antibiotic properties of bovine lactoferrin on *Helicobacter pylori*.' *Digestive Diseases and Sciences* December 43(12):2750-6.

Duff, M., and Ettarh, R. 2002. 'Crypt Cell Production Rate in the Small Intestine of the Zinc-Supplemented Mouse.' *Cells, Tissues, Organs* 172:21-28.

Elison, R.T. and Giehl, T.J. 1991. 'Killing of Gram-Negative Bacteria by Lactoferrin and Lysozyme.' *Journal of Clinical Investigation* 88(4):1080-1091.

Fertilizer Institute, The. 1982. *The Fertilizer Handbook.* 820 First Street, N.E. Suite 430, Washington, D.C. 20002.

Fiat, A.M., and Jolles, P. 1989. 'Caseins of various origins and biologically active casein peptides and oligosaccharides: structural and physiological aspects.' *Molecular and Cellular Biochemisty* May 4 87(1):5-30.

Gibson, G.R., Beaty, E.R., and Cummings, J.H. 1995.' Selective stimulation of bifidobacteria in the human colon by oligofructose and inulin.' *Gastroenterology* 108:975-82.

Golledge, C.L. and Riley, T.V. 1996. 'Natural therapy for infectious diseases.' *Medical Journal of Australia* 164:94-5.

Gordon, S., Todd, J., and Cohn, Z. 1974. 'In Vitro Synthesis and Secretion of Lysozyme of Mononuclear Phagocytes.' *Journal of Experimental Medicine* 139:1228.

Guslandi, M., Mezzi, G., Sorghi, M., and Testoni, P.A. 2000. '*Saccharomyces boulardii* in maintenance treatment of Crohn's disease.' *Digestive Diseases and Sciences* 45:1462-1464.

Hager, K., Felicetti, M., Seefried, G., and Platt, D. 1994. 'Fibrinogen and Aging.' *Aging* (Milano) 6:133-38.

Hill, G.M., Cromwell, G.L., Crenshaw, T.D., Dove, C.R., Ewan, R.C., Knabe, D.A., Lewis, A.J., Libal, G.W., Mahan, D.C., Shurson, G.C., Southern, L.L., and Veum, T.L. 2000. 'Growth promotion effects and plasma changes from feeding high dietary concentrations of zinc and copper to weanling pigs (regional study).' *Journal of Animal Science* 78:1010-1016.

Hosoi, T., Ametani, A., Kiuchi, K., and Kaminogawa, S. 2000. 'Improved growth and viability of lactobacilli in the presence of *Bacillus subtilis* (natto), catalase, or subtilisin.' *Canadian Journal of Microbiology* October 46(10):892-7.

Howarth, N.C., Huang, T.T., Roberts, S.B., and McCrory, M.A. 2005. 'Dietary fiber and fat are associated with excess weight in young and middle-aged US adults.' *Journal of the American Diet Association* September 105(9):1365-72.

Humphrey, B.D., Huang, N., and Klasing, K.C. 2002. 'Rice expressing lactoferrin and lysozyme has antibiotic-like properties when fed to chicks.' *Journal of Nutrition* 132:1214-1218.

Ilyinsky, O.B., Kozlova, M.V., Kondrikova, E.S., Kalentchuk, V.U., Titov, M.I., and Bespalova, Z.D. 1987. 'Effects of opioid peptides and naloxone on nervous tissue in culture.' *Neuroscience* August 22(2):719-35.

Imoto, T., Johnson, L., North, A., Phillips, D., and Rupley, J. (1972) 'Vertebrate Lysozymes.' *The Enzymes* Vol. 7, P. Boyer, Academic Press, New York.

Izadnia, F., Wong, C.T., and Kocoshis, S. (1998) 'Brewer's yeast and *Saccharomyces boulardii* both attenuate *Clostridium difficile*-induced colonic secretion in the rat.' *Digestive Diseases and Sciences* September 43(9):2055-60.

Jaffe, B.M. 1990. 'Serotonin in intestinal function. In Serotonin from cell biology to pharmacology and therapeutics.' Edited by Paoletti, R., Vanhoutte, P.M., Brunello, N., Maggi, F.M. London: Kluwer Academic Publishers; pp. 235-239.

Johns Hopkins Medical Institutions, The. 1997. The Johns Hopkins Microbiology Newsletter. Department of Pathology. July 28 16:28 Provided by Carmela

Groves, R.N., M.S., Chief, Division of Outbreak Investigation, Maryland Departent of Health and Mental Hygiene.

Katouli, M., Meliin, L., Jensen-Waern, M., Wallgren, P., and Mollby, R. 1999. 'The effect of zinc oxide supplementation on the stability of the intestinal flora with special reference to composition of coliforms in weaned pigs.' *Journal of Applied Microbiology* 87:564-573.

Lahov, E., and Regelson, W. 1996. 'Antibacterial and immunostimulating casein-derived substances from milk: casecidin, isracidin peptides.' *Food and Chemical Toxicology* January 34(1):131-45.

Lauer, D., Muller, R., Cott, C., Otto, A., Naumann, M., and Birkenmeier, G. 2001. 'Modulation of growth factor binding properties of alpha2-macroglobulin by enzyme therapy.' Institute of Biochemistry, University of Leipzig, Germany. *Cancer Chemotherapy and Pharmacology* July 47 (Suppl):S4-9.

Lauer, D., Reichenbach, A., and Birkenmeier, G. 2001. 'Alpha 2-macroglobulin-mediated degradation of amyloid beta 1- 42: a mechanism to enhance amyloid beta catabolism.' Institute of Biochemistry, University of Leipzig, Liebigstrasse 16 04103 Leipzig, Germany *Experimental Neurology* February 167(2):385-92.

Malkoski, M., Dashper, S.G., O'Brien-Simpson, N.M., Talbo, G., Macris, M., Cross, K.J., and Reynolds, E.C. 2001. 'Kappacin, a novel antibacterial peptide from bovine milk.' *Antimicrobial Agents and Chemotherapy* August 45(8):2309-15.

Masters, B.A., Kelly, E.J., Quaife, C.J., Brinster, R.L., and Palmiter, R.D. 1994. 'Targeted disruption of metallothionein I and II genes increases sensitivity to cadmium.' *Proceedings of the National Academy of Sciences* 91:584-588.

Mathlouthi, N., Lalles, J.P., Lepercq, P., Juste, C., and Larbier, M. 2002. 'Xylanase and beta-glucanase supplementation improve conjugated bile acid fraction in intestinal contents and increase villus size of small intestine wall in broiler chickens fed a rye-based diet.' *Journal of Animal Science* November 80(11):2773-9.

Meisel, H. 1997. 'Biochemical properties of regulatory peptides derived from milk proteins.' *Biopolymers* 43(2):119-28.

Molis, C., Flourie, B., Ouarne, F., Gailing, M.F., Lartigue, S., Guibert, A., Bornet, F., and Galmiche, J.P. 1996. 'Digestion, excretion, and energy value of fructooligosaccharides in healthy humans.' *American Journal of Clinical Nutrition* 64:324-8.

Mullins, J.E. and Fuentealba, I.C. 1998. 'Immunohistochemical detection of metallothionein in liver, duodenum and kidney after dietary copper-overload in rats.' *Histol Histopathology* July 13(3):627-33.

Pellegrini, A., Dettling, C., Thomas, U., and Hunziker, P. 2001. 'Isolation and characterization of four bactericidal domains in the bovine beta-lactoglobulin.' *Biochimica et Biophysica Acta* May 3 1526(2):131-40.

Proctor, V.A. and Cunningham, F.E. 1988. "The Chemistry of Lysozyme and its Use as a Food Preservative and a Pharmaceutical." *CRC Critical Reviews in Food Science and Nutrition* 26(4):359-395.

Quaife, C.J., Findley, S.D., Erickson, J.C., Froelic, G.J., Kelly, E.J., Zambrowicz, B.P., and Palmiter, R.D. 1994. 'Induction of a new metallothionein isoform

(MT-IV) occurs during differentiation of stratified squamous epithelia.' *Biochemistry* June *33*(23):7250-7259.

Recio, I., and Visser, S. 1999. 'Identification of two distinct antibacterial domains within the sequence of bovine alpha(s2)-casein.' *Biochimica et Biophysica Acta* August 5 *1428*(2-3):314-26.

Reid, L.D., and Hubbell, C.L. 1994. 'An assessment of the addiction potential of the opioid associated with milk.' *Journal of Dairy Science* March *77*(3):672-5.

Riordan, J.F., and Vallee, B.L. 1991. *Methods in Enzymology* Vol. 205 Academic Press Orlando, FL.

Roberfroid, M. 1993. 'Dietary fibre, inulin and oligofructose. A review comparing their physiological effects.' *Critical Reviews in Food Science and Nutrition* *33*:103-48.

Sakaguchi, M., Fujimori, T., Satoh, T., and Matsumura, E. 2001. 'Effects of beta-casomorphins on neuronal survival in culture of embryonic chick dorsal root ganglion neurons.' *Japanese Journal of Pharmacology* July *86*(3):363-5.

Samanya, M., and Yamauchi, K.E. 2002. 'Histological alterations of intestinal villi in chickens fed dried *Bacillus subtilis* var. *natto.*' *Comparative Biochemistry and Physiology Part A Molecular and Integrative Physiology* September *133*(1):95-104.

Spotts, R.A., Cervantes, L.A., Facteau, T.J., and Cand-Goyal, T. 1998. 'Control of brown rot and blue mold of sweet cherry with preharvest iprodione, postharvest *Cryptococcus infirmo-miniatus*, and modified atmosphere packaging.' *Plant Disease* *82*(10):1158-1160.

Szczurek, E.I., Bjornsson, C.S., and Taylor, C.G. 2001. 'Dietary zinc deficiency and repletion modulate metallothionein immunolocalization and concentration in small intestine and liver of rats.' *Journal of Nutrition* August *131*(8):2132-8.

Tomomatsu, H. 1994. 'Health effects of oligosaccharides.' *Food Technology* October:61-5.

Tran, C.D., Howarth, G.S., Coyle, P., Philcox, J.C., Rofe, A.M., and Butler, R.N. 2003. 'Dietary supplementation with zinc and a growth factor extract derived from bovine cheese whey improves methotrexate-damaged rat intestine.' *American Journal of Clinical Nutrition* 77:1296-1303.

Van den Heuvel, E.G., Muys, T., Van Dokkum, W., and Schaafsma, G. 1999. 'Oligofructose stimulates calcium absorption in adolescents.' *American Journal of Clinical Nutrition* 69:544-8.

Wood J.D., Alpers, D.H., and Andrews, P.L.R. 1999. 'Fundamentals of neurogastroenterology.' *Gut* 45(Suppl I):6-16.

Xu, Z.R., Hu, C.H., Xia, M.S., Zhan, X.A., and Wang, M.Q. 2003. 'Effects of dietary fructooligosaccharide on digestive enzyme activities, intestinal microflora and morphology of male broilers.' *Poultry Science* June *82*(6):1030-6.

Zucht, H.D., Raida, M., Adermann, K., Magert, H.J., and Forssmann, W.G. 1995. 'Casocidin-I: a casein-alpha s2 derived peptide exhibits antibacterial activity.' FEBS Letter September 25 *372*(2-3):185-8.

References for viral study with ViraStop

Bartsch, W. 1974. 'Proteolytic enzymes in the treatment of *Herpes zoster.' Der Informierte Arz* 2, 10, 1-7.

Billigmann, P. 1995. 'Enzyme therapy – An alternative in treatment of *Herpes zoster.* A controlled study of 192 patients.' *Fortschritte der Medizin 113*(4):43-48.

Billigmann, P.W. Wobe-Mugos® in the Therapy of *Herpes zoster.* Efficacy and Tolerance Study Number: MU-89105.

Jäger, H. 1990. 'Hydrolytic enzymes in the treatment of HIV infections.' *Allgemeinmedizin 19*:160-164.

Kabil, S., and Stauder, G. 1997. 'Oral enzyme therapy in hepatitis C patients.' *International Journal of Tissue Reactions* 1-2.

Kleine, M.W. 1997. 'Introduction to oral enzyme therapy and its use in *Varicella zoster* treatment.' *Ertl D. International Journal Tiss Reac* XIX (1/2), Abstracts of 7th Interscience World Conference on Inflammation, Antirheumatics, Analgesics, Immunomodulators, May 19-21, Geneva, Switzerland.

Korpan, M.I., Korpan, N.N., Tschekman, I.S., and Fialka, V. 1997. 'Mechanism of therapeutic efficacy of Wobenzym in the treatment of toxic hepatitis.' National Medical University, Kiev. *Dopovidi Nacionalnoi akademii nauk Ukrainy 9*:184-187.

Mendoza, A.G. 'Wobe-Mugos® E in the treatment of *Varicella zoster* infections.' Efficacy and Tolerance Study No.: MU-695502. Integrated final report according to ICH E3 guidelines. Instituto Dermatologico de Jalisco, Federalismo Norte # 3102, Atemajac, 44220 Guadalajara, Jalisco, Mexico.

Mikazans, I. 1997. 'Possibility to treat *Herpes zoster* using enzymes.' Department of Dermatology, Medical Academy of Latvia, Riga, Latvia. *Australasian Journal of Dermatology* 38(2). Abstracts of the 19th World Congress of Dermatology, 15-20 June, Sydney, Australia.

Mudrak, J., Bobak, L., and Sebova, I. 1997. 'Adjuvant therapy with hydrolytic enzymes in recurrent laryngeal papillomatosis.' *Acta Otolaryngologica Supplementum 527*:128-30. Department of Otorhinolaryngology, P.J. Safarik University Hospital, Kosice, Slovak Republic.

Mudrák, J., Koval, J., and Bobák, L. 2000. 'Systemic Enzymotherapy in Recurrent Laryngeal Papillomatosis - Our Five Year's Experience.' Epithelial tumours of the head and neck Proceedings, XXXIst Memorial Meeting for Professor Janez Plecnik, December 7-8, Ljubljana, Slovenia.

Mudrák, J., Sokol, L., Andrašovská, M., and Koval, J. 2000. 'Does Adjuvant Enzymotherapy Influence Recurrence of Schneiderian Papillomas?' Epithelial Tumours of the Head and Neck Proceedings XXXIst Memorial Meeting for Professor Janez Plecnik, 7-8. prosince, Ljubljana, Slovinsko.

Nikolaev, V.G., Matiasch, V.I., and Kononenko, V.V. 1998. 'Clinical use of Belosorb and Wobenzym in the Treatment of Viral Hepatitis B.' Presented at the conference 'Current approaches in infectology, epidemiology, and microbiology.' Kiev, Ukraine.

Patney, N.L., and Pachori, S. 1986. 'A Study of Serum Glycolytic Enzymes and Serum B Hepatitis in Relation to LIV.52 Therapy.' *The Medicine and Surgery* 4:9.

Pospíšilová, A., and Haklová, L. II. 1999. 'Clinical Experience with Systemic Enzyme Therapy in the Treatment of *Herpes zoster*.' Dermato-venerology clinic, Faculty Hospital Brno-Bohunice. Cesko-slovenská *Dermatologie* 74(1):17-20.

Scheef, W. (1987) 'Enzymtherapie, Lehrbuch der Naturheilverfahren.' *Hippokrates-Verlag* Bd. II, S. 95-103. (Hrgs. K.-Ch. Schimmer)

Stauder, G., and Kabil, S. 1997. 'Oral enzyme therapy in hepatitis C patients.' *International Journal of Immunotherapy* 3:153-158.

Stauder, G., and Kabil, S. 1997. 'Oral Enzyme Therapy in Hepatitis C patients.' *International Journal of Immunotherapy* XIII(3/4) 153-158. Mucos Pharma Clinical Research, Malvenweg 2, D-82538 Geretsried, Germany, and the Department of Hepatology, Gastroenterology & Infectious Diseases, Benha University Hospital, Cairo, Egypt.

Uffelmann, K. Wobe-Mugos® in the Therapy of *Herpes zoster* Infections. Efficacy and tolerance. Study Number: MU-88110. Leiter der Studie.

Immune system A2M

Castell, J.V., Friedrich, G., Kuhn, C.S., and Poppe, G.E. 1997. 'Intestinal absorption of undegraded proteins in men: presence of bromelain in plasma after oral intake.' *American Journal of Physiology* 273(1 Pt 1):G139-46.

Desser, L., Holomanova, D., Zavadova, E., Pavelka, K., Mohr, T., and Herbacek, I. 2001. 'Oral therapy with proteolytic enzymes decreases excessive TGF-beta levels in human blood.' Institute of Cancer Research, University of Vienna, Austria. *Cancer Chemotherapy and Pharmacology* July 47(Suppl):S10-5.

Lauer, D., Muller, R., Cott, C., Otto, A., Naumann, M., and Birkenmeier, G. 2001. 'Modulation of growth factor binding properties of alpha2-macroglobulin by enzyme therapy.' Institute of Biochemistry, University of Leipzig, Germany. *Cancer Chemotherapy and Pharmacology* July 47(Suppl):S4-9.

Lauer, D., Reichenbach, A., and Birkenmeier, G. 2001. 'Alpha 2-macroglobulin-mediated degradation of amyloid beta 1—42: a mechanism to enhance amyloid beta catabolism.' Institute of Biochemistry, University of Leipzig, Liebigstrasse 16, 04103 Leipzig, Germany. *Experimental Neurology* February 167(2):385-92.

Strickland, D.K, and Ranganathan, S. 2003. 'Diverse role of LDL receptor-related protein in the clearance of proteases and in signaling.' Department of Vascular Biology, Jerome H. Holland Laboratory for the Biomedical Sciences, American Red Cross, Rockville, MD, USA. *Journal of Thrombosis and Haemostasis* July 1(7):1663-70.

Further References

www.enzymedica.com Enzymedica enzyme company
www.enzymestuff.com Enzyme information, author's website
www.enzymeuniversity.com Enzyme information
www.theramedix.net Professional enzyme line company
www.transformationenzymes.com Professional enzyme line company
www.wobenzym.com Enzyme company

Bohager, T. 2006. *Enzymes: What the Experts Know!* One World Press. Prescott, Arizona.

Brady, N., and Weil, R. 2001. *The Nature and Properties of Soils.* 13th edition. Prentice Hall. Upper Saddle River, New Jersey.

Cichoke, A. 1994 *Enzymes and Enzyme Therapy: How to Jump-Start Your Way to Lifelong Good Health.* Keats Publishing. Los Angeles, California.

Cutler, E. 2005. *MicroMiracles: Discover the Healing Power of Enzymes.* Rodale Press. Emmaus, Pennsylvania.

Fallon, Sally, Mary G. Enig, and Kim Waters. 1999, 2nd edition. *Nourishing Traditions: The Cookbook that Challenges Politically Correct Nutrition and the Diet Dictocrats.* New Trends Publishing, Incorporated. Winona Lake, IN.

Fuller, D. 1998. *The Healing Power of Enzymes.* Forbes Custom Publishing. New York, New York.

Gates, Donna. 1996. *Body Ecology.* B.E.D. Publications Atlanta, Georgia.

Gershon, M. 1998. *The Second Brain: The Scientific Basis of Gut Instinct and a Groundbreaking New Understanding of Nervous Disorders of the Stomach and Intestines.* HarperCollins Publishers Inc. New York, New York.

Gottschall, E. 1994. *Breaking the Vicious Cycle: Intestinal Health Through Diet.* Kirkton Press. Ontario, Canada.

Guyton, A., and Hall, J. *Textbook of Medical Physiology.* 10th edition. W.B. Saunders Company. Philadelphia, Pennsylvania.

Hersey, J. 1996. *Why Can't My Child Behave?* Pear Tree Press, Inc., Alexandria, Virginia.

Howell, E. 1985. *Enzyme Nutrition: The Food Enzyme Concept.* Avery Publishing. Wayne, New Jersey.

Howell, E. 1994. *Food Enzymes for Health and Longevity.* Lotus Press. Twin Lakes, Wisconsin.

In Salinas, A.F., and Hanna, G. M. *Immune Complexes and Human Cancer,* Vol 15. Plenum Press. New York, New York. eds.

King, J.E. 2000. *Mayo Clinic on Digestive Health.* Mayo Foundation for Medical Education and Research. Rochester, Minnesota.

Lipski, E. 2006. *Digestive Wellness for Children.* Basic Health Publications. Laguna Beach, California.

Lipski, E. 1996. *Digestive Wellness.* Keats Publishing. Los Angeles, California.

Lopez, D.A., Williams, M., and Miehlke. 1994. *Enzymes – The Fountain of Life.* The Neville Press. Charleston, South Carolina.

Rapp, D. 1991. *Is This Your Child?* William Morrow and Company. New York, New York.

Tisdale, S., Werner, N., and Beaton, W. 2004. *Soil Fertility and Fertilizers - An Introductionto Nutrient Management.* 7th edition. Prentice Hall. Upper Saddle River, New Jersey.

Thompson, W.G. 1989. *Gut Reactions: Understanding Symptoms of the Digestive Tract.* Plenum Press. New York, New York.

Wolf, M., and Ransberger, K. 1972. *Enzyme Therapy.* New York. Vantage Press. out of print.

There are many good books available on food additives, food and chemical sensitivities/intolerances/allergies, nutrition, and effects on behavior as well.

Groups providing information on digestive health and nutrition

American Academy of Family Physicians (AAFP)
11400 Tomahawk Creek Parkway
Leawood, KS 66211-2672
Toll free: 800-274-2237

American Dietetic Association (ADA) recommends
120 South Riverside Plaza, Suite 2000
Chicago, Illinois 60606-6995
Phone: 800/877-1600
www.eatright.org

Cystic Fibrosis Foundation
6931 Arlington Road, Bethesda, Maryland 20814
(301) 951-4422 or (800) 344-4823
www.cff.org, info@cff.org

International Foundation for Functional Gastrointestinal Disorders
P.O. Box 170864, Milwaukee, WI 53217
Phone: 1–888–964–2001
Email: iffgd@iffgd.org
www.iffgd.org

National Institute of Diabetes and Digestive and Kidney Diseases (NIDDK), National
  Institutes of Health
2 Information Way, Bethesda, MD 20892–3570
Phone: 1–800–891–5389
Email: nddic@info.niddk.nih.gov

U.S. National Library of Medicine,
8600 Rockville Pike, Bethesda, MD 20894
www.nlm.nih.gov

Weston A. Price Foundation
Phone: 202.363.4394, www.westonaprice.org

Worthington Biochemical Corporation
730 Vassar Ave, Lakewood, NJ, 08701
(732) 942-1660, 1-800-445-9603

Even Further References

Carver, J.D. 2003. 'Advances in nutritional modifications of infant formulas.' *American Journal of Clinical Nutrition* June 77(6):1550S-1554S.

Clare, D.A., Catignani, G.L., and Swaisgood, H.E. 2003. 'Biodefense properties of milk: the role of antimicrobial proteins and peptides.' *Current Pharmaceutical Design* 9(16):1239-55.

Dohler, J.R., and Nebermann, L. 2002. 'Bovine colostrum in oral treatment of enterogenic endotoxaemia in rats.' *Critical Care* December 6(6):536-9.

Isaacs, C.E, Litov, R.E., and Thormar, H. 1995. 'Antimicrobial activity of lipids added to human milk, infant formula, and bovine milk.' *Journal of Nutritional Biochemistry* July 6(7):362-366.

Isaacs, C.E., Pullar, Kat R., and Kascsak, R. 2001. 'Development of a topical vaginal microbicide: lessons learned from human milk.' *Advances in Experimental Medicine and Biology* 501:223-32.

Hamosh, M. 1998. 'Protective function of proteins and lipids in human milk.' *Biology of the Neonate* 74(2):163-76.

Kushnareva, M.V., Keshishian, E.S., and Soboleva, S.V. 1995. 'The efficacy of using an immune lactoglobulin preparation for correcting intestinal dysbacteriosis in newborn infants.' *Zhurnal Mikrobiologii, Epidemiologii, i Immunobiologii* March-April (2):101-4.

Playford, R.J., Macdonald, C.E., and Johnson, W.S. 2000. 'Colostrum and milk-derived peptide growth factors for the treatment of gastrointestinal disorders.' *American Journal of Clinical Nutrition* July 72(1):5-14.

Van der Strate, B.W., Beljaars, L., Molema, G., Harmsen, M.C., and Meijer, D.K. 2001. 'Antiviral activities of lactoferrin.' *Antiviral Research* December 52(3):225-39.

Van Hooijdonk, A.C., Kussendrager, K.D., and Steijns, J.M. 2000. 'In vivo antimicrobial and antiviral activity of components in bovine milk and colostrum involved in non-specific defence.' *British Journal of Nutrition* Nov 84(Suppl 1):S127-34.

Research on enzymes and intestinal permeability (leaky gut)

Ambrus, J.L., Lassman, H.B., and DeMarchi, J.J. 1967. 'Absorption of exogenous and endogenous proteolytic enzymes.' *Clinical Pharmacology and Therapeutics* 8:362-8.

Amoss, M., et al. 1972. 'Release of gonadotrophins by oral administration of synthetic LRF or a tripeptidle fragment of LRF.' *Journal of Clinical Endocrinology and Metabolism* 35:135-177.*

Andre, C., et al. 1974. 'Interference of oral immunization with the intestinal absorption of heterologous albumin.' *European Journal of Immunology* 4:701-704.*

Avakian, S. 1964. 'Further studies on the absorption of chymotrypsin.' *Clinical Pharmacology and Therapeutics* 5:712-5.

Bergkvist, R., and Svard, P.C. 1964. 'Studies on the thrombolytic effect of a protease from *Aspergillus oryzae*.' *Acta Physiologica Scandanavica* 60:363-371.

Bjarnason, I., et al. 1984. 'Intestinal permeability in celiac sprue, dermatitis herpetiformis, schizophrenia, and atopic eczema.' *Gastroenterology* 86:1029.*

Bockman, D.E., and Winborm, W.B. 1966. 'Light and electron microscopy of intestinal ferritin absorption: Observations in sensitized and non-sensitized hamsters.' *Anatomical Record* 155:603-622.

Campbell, C.A., Forrest, J., and Muscgrove, C. 1994. 'High-strength pancreatic enzyme supplements and large-bowel stricture in cystic fibrosis.' *Lancet* 343:109-10 [letter].

Cichoke, A.J. 1995. 'The effect of systemic enzyme therapy on cancer cells and the immune system.' *Townsend Letter for Doctors and Patients* November 30-2 [review].

Dannaeus, A., et al. 1979. 'Intestinal uptake of ovalbumin in malabsorption and food allergy in relation to serum IgG antibody and orally administrated sodium chromoglycate.' *Clin. Allergy* 9:263-270.*

Deitrick, R.E. 1965. 'Oral proteolytic enzymes in the treatment of athletic injuries: a double-blind study.' *Pennsylvania Med J* October 35-7.*

DiMagno, E.P., et al. 1973. 'Relations between pancreatic enzyme outputs and malabsorption in severe pancreatic insufficiency.' *New England Journal of Medicine* 228:813-815.*

Ferguson, A. and Caldwell, F. 1972. 'Precipitins to dietary proteins in serum and upper GI secretion of coeliac children.' *British Medical Journal* 1:75-77.

Fitzgerald, D.E., et al. 1979. 'Relief of chronic arterial obstruction using intravenous brinase.' *Scandinavian Journal of Thoracic and Cardiovascular Surgery* 13:327-332.*

Fitzgerald, D. and Frisch, E.P. 1973. 'Relief of chronic peripheral artery obstruction by intravenous brinase.' *Irish Med. Ass.* 66:3.*

Frisch, E.P. and Blomback, M. 1979. 'Blood coagulation studies in patients treated with brinase.' In: Progress in Chemical Fibrinolysis and Thrombolysis. Vol. IV, J.F. Davidson (Ed.), Edinburgh: Churchill-Livingstone, pp. 184-187.

Frisch, E. P., et al. 1975. 'Dosage of i. v. brinase in man based on brinase inhibitor capacity and coagulation studies.' *Angiology* 26:557.*

Gardner, M.L.G. 1988. 'Gastrointestinal absorption of intact proteins.' *Annual Review of Nutrition* 8:329-350.

Gardner, M. L. G. 1984. 'Intestinal assimilation of intact peptides and proteins from the diet - A neglected field?' *Biol. Review* 59:289-331.*

Gonzalez, N.J. and Isaacs, L.L. 1999. 'Evaluation of pancreatic proteolytic enzyme treatment of adenocarcinoma of the pancreas, with nutrition and detoxification support.' *Nutrition and Cancer 33*:117-24.

Griffin, S. M., *et al*. 1989. 'Acid resistant lipase as replacement therapy in chronic exocrine insufficiency: a study in dogs.' *Gut* 30:1012-1015.

Gullo, L. 1993. 'Indication for pancreatic enzyme treatment in non-pancreatic digestive diseases.' *Digestion 54*(Suppl 2):43-7.

Hamilton, I., *et al*. 1993. 'Small intestinal permeability in dermatological disease.' *Quarterly Journal of Medicine 56*:559-567.*

Heatley, R.V., *et al*. 1993. 'Inflammatory bowel disease, In Gut Defenses in Clinical Practice.' M.S. Losowsky and R.V. Heatley, eds., Churchill Livingstone, Edinburgh, pp. 225-277.*

Heinrich, J., Balleisen, L., Schulte, H., Assmann, G., and Van de Loo, J. 1994. 'Fibrinogen and factor VII in the prediction of coronary risk.' *Arteriosclerosis and Thrombosis 14*:54-59.

Hemmings, W.A., and Williams, E.W. 1978. 'Transport of large breakdown products of dietary protein through the gut wall.' *Gut 19*:715-723.

Husby, S., *et al*. 1987. 'Passage of dietary antigens into the blood of children with coeliac disease: Quantification and size distribution of absorbed antigens.' *Gut 28*:1062-1072

Husby, S., *et al*. 1986. 'Passage of undergrade dietary antigen into the blood of healthy adults: further characterization of the kinetics of uptake and the size distribution of the antigen.' *Scandanavian Journal of Immunology 24*:447-455.

Izaka, K., Yamada, M., Kawano, T., and Suyama, T. 1972. 'Gastrointestinal absorption and anti-inflammatory effect of bromelain.' *Japanese Journal of Pharmacology 22*:519-34.

Jackson, P.G., *et al*. 1981. 'Intestinal permeability in patients with eczema and food allergy.' *Lancet 1*:1285-1286.*

Jacobson, I., *et al*. 1986. 'Human beta-lactalbumin as a marker of macromolecular absorption.' *Gut 27*:1029-1034.*

Jones, R., Franklin, K., Spicer, R., and Berry, J. 1995. 'Colonic strictures in children with cystic fibrosis on low-strength pancreatic enzymes.' *Lancet 346*:499-500 [letter].

Larson, L.J., *et al*. 1988. 'Properties of the complex between alpha-2-macro-globulin and brinase, a proteinase from *Aspergillus oryzae* with thrombolytic effect, thrombosis.' *Research 49*:55-68.*

Laskowski, M., *et al*. 1958. 'Effect of trypsin inhibitor on passage of insulin across the intestinal barrier.' *Science 127*:1115-1116.*

Layer, P., and Groger, G. 1993. 'Fate of pancreatic enzymes in the human intestinal lumen in health and pancreatic insufficiency.' *Digestion 54*(Suppl 2):10-4.

Liebow, C. and Rothman, S.S. 1975. 'Enteropancreatic circulation of digestive enzymes.' *Science 189*:472-474.

Loehry, C. A., *et al*. 1970. 'Permeability of the small intestine to substances of different molecular weight.' *Gut 11*:446-470.*

Lund, F., *et al.* 1975. 'Thrombolytic treatment with i.v. brinase in advance arterial obliterative disease.' *Angiology 26*:534.*

Kiesslling, H. and Svenson, R. 1970. 'Influence of an enzyme from *Aspergillus oryzae*, Protease 1, on some components of the fibrinolytic system.' *Acta Chemica Scandanavica 24*:569-579.

Kleine, M.W., Stauder, G.M, and Beese, E.W. 1995. 'The intestinal absorption of orally administered hydrolytic enzymes and their effects in the treatment of acute *Herpes zoster* as compared with those of oral acyclovir therapy.' *Phytomedicine 2*:7-15.

Mackie, R.D., *et al.* 1981. 'Malabsorption of starch in pancreatic sufficiency.' *Gastroenterology 80*:1220.*

McCann, M. 1993. 'Pancreatic enzyme supplement for treatment of multiple food allergies.' *Annals of Allergy 71*:269.

McCarthy, C.F. 1976. 'Nutritional defects in patients with malabsorption.' *Proceedings of the Nutrition Society 35*:37-40.

Menzies, I.S. 1984. 'Transmucosal passage of inert molecules in health and disease.' In Intestinal Absorption and Secretion, E. Skadhauge and K Heintze, eds., MTP Press, Lancaster, pp. 527-543.

Milla, C.E., Wielinski, C.L., and Warwick, W.J. 1994. 'High-strength pancreatic enzymes.' *Lancet 343*:599 [letter].

Moretti, M., Bertoli, E., Bulgarelli, S., Testoni, C., Guffanti, E.E., Marchioni, C.F., and Braga, P.C. 1993. 'Effects of seaprose on sputum biochemical components in chronic bronchitic patients: a double-blind study vs placebo.' *International Journal of Clinical Pharmacology Research 13*(5):275-80.

Nakamura, T., Tandoh, Y., Terada, A., *et al.* (1998) 'Effects of high-lipase pancreatin on fecal fat, neutral sterol, bile acid, and short-chain fatty acid excretion in patients with pancreatic insufficiency resulting from chronic pancreatitis.' *International Journal of Pancreatology 23*:63-70.*

Oades, P.J., Bush, A., Ong, P.S., and Brereton, R.J. 1994. 'High-strength pancreatic enzyme supplements and large-bowel stricture in cystic fibrosis.' *Lancet 343*:109 [letter].

Oelgoetz, A.W., Oelgoetz, P.A., and Wittenkind, J. 1935. 'The treatment of food allergy and indigestion of pancreatic origin with pancreatic enzymes.' *American Journal of Digestive Diseases Nutr 2*:422-6.

Ormistron, B.J. 1972. 'Clinical effects of TRH and TSH after i.v. and oral administration in normal volunteers and patients with thyroid disease.' In Thytropin Releasing Hormone (Frontiers of Hormone) Research, Vol. 1, R. Hall, *et al*, eds., Karger, Basel pp. 45-52.

Patel, R.S., Johlin, F.C. Jr., and Murray, J.A. 1999. 'Celiac disease and recurrent pancreatitis.' *Gastrointestinal Endoscopy 50*:823-7.

Phelan, J.J., *et al.* 1977. 'Coeliac disease: The abolition of gliadin toxicity by enzymes from *Aspergillus niger*.' *Clin. Sci. Molec. Med. 53*:35-43.*

Powell, C.J. 1999. 'Pancreatic enzymes and fibrosing colonopathy.' *Lancet 354*:251 [letter].

Roschlau, H.E., and Fisher, A.M. 1966. 'Thrombolytic therapy with local perfusions of CA-7 (fibrinolytic enzyme from *Aspergillus oryzae*) in the dog.' *Angiology* 17:670-682.

Seligman, B. 1962. 'Bromelain: an anti-inflammatory agent.' *Angiology* 13:508-10.

Siefert, J., et al. 'Mucosal permeation of Macromolecules and particles.' See Ref 31, pp. 505-513.*

Shorter, R.G., et al. 1972. 'A working hypothesis for the etiology and pathogenesis of nonspecific inflammatory bowel disease.' *American Journal of Digestive Diseases* 17:1024-1032.*

Stevens, J.C., Maguiness, K.M., Hollingsworth, J., et al. 1998. 'Pancreatic enzyme supplementation in cystic fibrosis patients before and after fibrosing colonopathy.' *Journal of Pediatric Gastroenterology and Nutrition* 26:80-4.*

Suarez, F., Levitt, M.D., Adshead, J., and Barkin, J.S. 1999. 'Pancreatic supplements reduce symptomatic response of healthy subjects to a high fat meal.' *Digestive Diseases and Sciences* 44:1317-21.

Sumi, H., Hamada, H., Tsushima, H., Mihara, H., and Muraki, H. 1987. 'Novel fibrinolytic enzyme (nattokinase) in the vegetable cheese Natto; a typical and popular soybean food in the Japanese diet.' *Experientia* October 3(10):1110-1.

Sumi, H., Hamada, H., Nakanishi, K., and Hiratani, H. 1990. 'Enhancement of the fibrinolytic activity in plasma by oral administration of nattokinase.' *Acta Haematologica* 84(3):139-43.

Suzuki, Y., Kondo, K., Maeda, T., Matsumoto, Y., Otsuguro, K., Tsukamoto, Y., Umemura, K., Urano, T., and Zhao, B. (2003) 'Dietary supplementation of fermented soybean, natto, suppresses intimal thickening and modulates the lysis of mural thrombi after endothelial injury in rat femoral artery.' *Life Sciences* 73:1289-1298.

Suzuki, Y., Kondo, K., Ichise, H., Tsukamoto, Y., Urano, T., and Umemura, K. 2003. 'Dietary supplementation with fermented soybeans suppresses intimal thickening.' *Nutrition* 19(3):261-4.

Taylor, C.J., Hillel, P.G., Ghosal, S., et al. 1999. 'Gastric emptying and intestinal transit of pancreatic enzyme supplements in cystic fibrosis.' *Archives of Disease in Childhood* 80:149-52.*

Udall, J.N., and Walker, W.A. 1982. 'The physiologic and pathologic basis for the transport of macromolecule's across the intestinal tract.' *Journal of Pediatric Gastroentarology and Nutrition* 295-301.

Vanhove, P., et al. 1979. 'Action of brinase on human fibrinogen and plasminogen.' *Journal of Thrombosis and Haemostasis* 42:571-581.*

Verhaege, R., et al. 1979. 'Clinical trial of brinase and anticoagulants as a method of treatment for advanced limb ischemia.' *European Journal of Clinical Pharmacology* 16165-170.*

Verstraefe, M., and Verhaege, R. 1977. 'Clinical study if brinase, a proteolytic enzyme from *Aspergillus oryzae*.' 19th Annual Congr. Intern,. Coll. Angiology, Dublin, Ireland.

Walker, W.A. 1975. 'Antigen absorption from the small intestine and gastrointestinal disease.' *Pediatric Clinics of North America* 22:731-746.

Warshaw, A.L., et al. 1974. 'Protein uptake by the intestine: Evidence for absorption of intact macromolecules.' Gastroenterology 66:987-992.*

Wolf, J.L., et al. 1981. 'Intestinal M cells: A pathway for entry of retrovirus into the host.' Science 212:471-472.*

Wolf, M., and Ransberger, K. 1972. Enzyme Therapy New York: Vantage Press, 135-220 [review].

Research enzymes and bacteria

Ivaniyta, L.I., Ivaniyta, S.O., Kornatskaya, A.G., Belis, N.I., and Kondratiyk*. 1998. 'Systemic enzyme therapy in the treatment of chronic salpingitis and infertility.' Institute of Pediatrics, Obstetrics, and Gynecology, Ukraine Farmatsevtychnyi Zhurnal (Kiev) 2:89-92.*

Konno, K., Hirayama, C., Nakamura, M., Tateishi, K., Tamura, Y., Hattori, M., and Kohno, K. 2004. 'Papain protects papaya trees from herbivorous insects: role of cysteine proteases in latex.' Plant Journal February 37(3):370-8.

Protsenko, T.V. 1998. 'Systemic enzyme therapy in dermatology and venerology: perspectives of its use.' State Medical Uiniversity, Donetsk, Ukraine Zurnal dermatologii i venerologii 2(6):12-13.

Shahid, S.K., Turakhia, N.H., Kundra, M., Shanbag, P., Daftary, G.V., and Schiess, W. 2002. 'Efficacy and safety of phlogenzym—a protease formulation, in sepsis in children.' LTMMC and LTMG Hospital and Medical College, Mumbai. Journal of the Association of Physicians of India April 50:527-31.

Sukhikh, G.T., Loginova, N.S., Faizullin, L.Z., Zdanov, A.V., Malinina, E.V, and Bozedomov, V.A. 1997. 'The use of WOBENZYM® to facilitate interferon synthesis in the treatment of chronic urogenital chlamydiosis.' International Journal of Immunotherapy XIII(3/4) 131-133. International Journal of Tissue Reactions XIX (1/2), 1997 - abstracts of 7th Interscience World Conference on Inflammation, Antirheumatics, Analgesics, Immunomodulators, May 19-21, Geneva, Switzerland.

Veldová, Z., Martínková, R., and Maderová, S. 1999. 'Use of Phlogenzym® in the treatment of secretory otitis in the outpatient practice.' Audiocentrum Praha Congress of the Czech Society of Otorhinolaryngology and Surgery of Head and Neck, September 9-11, Hradec Králové, Czech Republic.

Research on nattokinase

Chang, C.T., Fan, M.H., Kuo, F.C., and Sung, H.Y. 2000. 'Potent fibrinolytic enzyme from a mutant of Bacillus subtilis IMR-NK1.' Journal of Agriculture and Food Chemistry August 48(8):3210-6.

Chiang, C.J., Chen, H.C., Chao, Y.P., and Tzen, J.T. 2005. 'Efficient system of artificial oil bodies for functional expression and purification of recombinant nattokinase in Escherichia coli.' Journal of Agriculture and Food Chemistry June 15 53(12):4799-804.

Fujita, M., Hong, K., Ito, Y., Fujii, R., Kariya, K., and Nishimuro, S. 1995. 'Thrombolytic effect of nattokinase on a chemically induced thrombosis model in rat.' *Biological and Pharmaceutical Bulletin* October *18*:1387-91.

Fujita, M., Hong, K., Ito, Y., Misawa, S., Takeuchi, N., Kariya, K., and Nishimuro, S. 1995. 'Transport of nattokinase across the rat intestinal tract.' *Biological and Pharmaceutical Bulletin* *18*:1194-6.

Fujita, M., Nomura, K., Hong, K., Ito, Y., Asada, A., and Nishimuro, S. 1993. 'Purification and characterization of a strong fibrinolytic enzyme (nattokinase) in the vegetable cheese natto, a popular soybean fermented food in Japan.' *Biochemical and Biophysical Research Communications* December *197*(3):1340-7.

Guo, J., Sun, Y., and Su, Y. 2002. 'Preparation of natto and its function in health care.' *Zhong Yao Cai* January *25*(1):61-4.

Institute of Health Sciences. 2002. 'Prevent Heart Attack and Stroke with Potent Enzyme that Dissolves Deadly Blood Clots in Hours.' *Health Sciences Institute Newsletter* March.

Kim, W., Choi, K., Kim, Y., Park, H., Choi, J., Lee, Y., Oh, H., Kwon, I., and Lee, S. 1996. 'Purification and characterization of a fibrinolytic enzyme produced from *Bacillus* sp. strain CK 11-4 screened from Chungkook-Jang.' *Applied and Environmental Microbiology* July *62*(7):2482-8. ·

Ko, J.H, Yan, J.P, Zhu, L, and Qi, Y.P. 2004. 'Identification of two novel fibrinolytic enzymes from *Bacillus subtilis* QK02.' *Comparative Biochemistry and Physiology C Toxicology and Pharmacology* January *137*(1):65-74.

Liu, B.Y., and Song, H.Y. 2002. 'Molecular cloning and expression of nattokinase gene in *Bacillus subtilis.*' Sheng Wu Hua Xue Yu Sheng Wu Wu Li Xue Bao (Shanghai) May *34*(3):338-40.

Liu, J.G., Xing, J.M., Chang, T.S., and Liu, H.Z. (2005) 'Purification of nattokinase by reverse micelles extraction from fermentation broth: effect of temperature and phase volume ratio.' *Bioprocess and Biosystems Engineering* December *8*:1-7.

Maeda, H., Mizutani, O., Yamagata, Y., Ichishima, E., and Nakajima, T. 2001. 'Alkaline-resistance model of subtilisin ALP I, a novel alkaline subtilisin.' *Journal of Biochemistry* (Tokyo) May *129*(5):675-82.

Peng, Y., Huang, Q., Zhang, R.H., and Zhang, Y.Z. 2003. 'Purification and characterization of a fibrinolytic enzyme produced by *Bacillus amyloliquefaciens* DC-4 screened from douchi, a traditional Chinese soybean food.' *Comparative Biochemistry and Physiology B Biochemistry and Molecular Biology* January *134*(1):45-52.

Takano, A., Hirata, A., Ogasawara, K., Sagara, N., Inomata, Y., Kawaji, T., and Tanihara, H. 2006. 'Posterior Vitreous Detachment Induced by Nattokinase (Subtilisin NAT): A Novel Enzyme for Pharmacologic Vitreolysis.' *Investigative Ophthalmology and Visual Science* May *47*(5):2075-9.

Urano, T., Ihara, H., Umemura, K., Suzuki, Y., Oike, M., Akita, S., Tsukamoto, Y., Suzuki, I., and Takada, A. 2001. 'The profibrinolytic enzyme subtilisin NAT purified from *Bacillus subtilis* cleaves and inactivates plasminogen activator inhibitor type 1.' *Journal of Biological Chemistry* July *276*(27):24690-6.

Zheng, Z.L., Ye, M.Q., Zuo, Z.Y., Liu, Z.G., Tai, K.C., and Zou, G.L. 2006. 'Probing the importance of hydrogen bonds in the active site of the subtilisin nattokinase by site-directed mutagenesis and molecular dynamics simulation.' *Biochemical Journal* May 1 *395*(3):509-15.

Zheng, Z., Zuo, Z., Liu, Z., Tsai, K., Liu, A., and Zou, G. 2005. 'Construction of a 3D model of nattokinase , a novel fibrinolytic enzyme from *Bacillus natto* - A novel nucleophilic catalytic mechanism for nattokinase.' *Journal of Molecular Graphics and Modelling* 23:373-380.

Research studies on seaprose

Antonelli, A., Cimino, A., Cimino, A., Di Girolamo, A., Filippi, P., Filippin, S., Galetti, G., Marchiori, C., Marcucci, L., Mira, E., et al. 1993. 'The treatment of ENT phlogosis: seaprose S vs. nimesulide.' *Acta Otorhinolaryngologica Italica* 13(Suppl 39):1-16. *

Banchini, G., Scaricabarozzi, I., Montecorboli, U., Ceccarelli, A., Chiesa, F., Ditri, L., Mazzer, G., Moroni, R., Viola, M., Roggia, F., et al. 1993. 'Double-blind study of nimesulide in divers with inflammatory disorders of the ear, nose and throat.' *Drugs* 46(Suppl 1):100-2.*

Bracale, G. and Selvetella, L. 1996. 'Clinical study of the efficacy of and tolerance to seaprose S in inflammatory venous disease. Controlled study versus serratio-peptidase.' *Minerva Cardioangiologica* October 44(10):515-24.

Braga, P.C., Moretti, M., Piacenza, A., Montoli, C.C., and Guffanti, E.E. 1993. 'Effects of seaprose on the rheology of bronchial mucus in patients with chronic bronchitis. A double-blind study vs placebo.' *International Journal of Clinical Pharmacology Research* 13(3):179-85.

Braga, P.C., Piatti, G., Grasselli, G., Casali, W., Beghi, G., and Allegra, L. 1992. 'The influence of seaprose on erythromycin penetration into bronchial mucus in bronchopulmonary infections.' *Drugs Under Experimental and Clinical Research* 18(3):105-11.

Braga, P. C., Rampoldi, C., Ornaghi, A., Caminiti, G., Beghi, G., and Allegra, L. 1990. 'In vitro rheological assessment of mucolytic activity induced by seaprose.' *Pharmacological Research* September-October 22(5):611-7.

Dindelli, M., Potenza, M. T., Candotti, G., Frigerio, L., and Pifarotti, G. 1990. 'Clinical effectiveness and safety of Seaprose S in the treatment of complications of puerperal surgical wounds.' *Minerva Ginecologica* July-August 42(7-8):313-5.

Fossati, A. 1999. 'Anti-inflammatory effects of seaprose-S on various inflammation models.' *Drugs Under Experimental and Clinical Research* 25(6):263-70.

Giorgetti, P.L., Bortolani, E.M., Morbidelli, A., Vandone, P.L., Ghilardi, G., Mattioli, A., and Giordanengo, F. 1990. 'Use of a new anti-inflammatory drug in the treatment of varicophlebitis of the lower limbs.' *Minerva Chirurgica* June 30 45(12):883-6.

Ito, F., Uchida, H., Konishiike, J., Yamazaki, M., and Yamamoto, Y. 1973. 'Clinical examination of proteolytic enzyme preparation, seaprose S, in liquefaction of the sputum: comparison using a double blind test. *Nippon Rinsho* July 31(7):2339-44.

Kase, Y., Seo, H., Oyama, Y., Sakata, M., Tomoda, K., Takahama, K., Hitoshi, T., Okano, Y., and Mayata, T. 1982. 'A new method for evaluating mucolytic expectorant activity and its application. II. Application to two proteolytic enzymes, serratiopeptidase and seaprose.' *Arzneimittelforschung* 32(4):374-8.

Kidaand, J., and Kano, K. 1967. 'Effect of oral administration of a mold protease on the concentration of antibiotics in rat bronchial wash.' *

Korzus, E., Luisetti, M., and Travis, J. 1994. 'Interactions of alpha-1-antichymotrypsin, alpha-1-proteinase inhibitor, and alpha-2-macroglobulin with the fungal enzyme, seaprose.' *Biological Chemistry Hoppe Seyler* May *375*(5):335-41.

Luisetti, M., Piccioni, P.D., Dyne, K., Donnini, M., Bulgheroni, A., Pasturenzi, L., Donnetta, A.M., and Peona, V. 1991. 'Some properties of the alkaline proteinase from *Aspergillus melleus.' International Journal of Tissue Reactions 13*(4):187-92.

Tanimoto, T., Fukuda, H., and Kawamura, J. 1983. 'On the quality of enzyme preparation (IV). Seaprose S preparation.' *Eisei Shikenjo Hokoku* (101):88-91.

Research on serratiopeptidase

Alessandrini, A., Ferrari, D., Bastianon, A., and Maccagno, A. 1985. 'Granulated feprazone in acute inflammatory pathology of the bronchial tree. Study in comparison to a serratiopeptidase.' *La Clinica Terapeutica* May *113*(4):275-80.

Aratani, H., Kono, S., and Yamanaka, Y. 1974. 'Fundamental studies on the distribution of sulfobenzylpenicillin. Effect of serratiopeptidase (author's transl).' *Japanese Journal of Antibiotics* June *27*(3):271-8.

Aratani, H., Tateishi, H., and Negita, S. 1979. 'Studies on in vivo activity of antibiotics in experimental pneumonia in rats. I. Combination of ciclacillin and serratiopeptidase (author's transl).' *Japanese Journal of Antibiotics* August *32*(8):806-11.

Aratani, H., Tateishi, H., and Negita, S. 1980. 'Studies on the distributions of antibiotics in the oral tissues: Experimental staphylococcal infection in rats, and effect of serratiopeptidase on the distributions of antibiotics.' *Japanese Journal of Antibiotics* May *33*(5):623-35.

Bracale, G., and Selvetella, L. 1996. 'Clinical study of the efficacy of and tolerance to seaprose S in inflammatory venous disease. Controlled study versus serratiopeptidase.' *Minerva Cardioangiologica* October *44*(10):515-24.

Bruno, E., Porcellini, A., and Farronato, G.P. 1986. 'Clinical study of a new oral anti-inflammatory: Zami 642.' *Dental Cadmos* October *54*(15):81-3.

Bucci, E., Mignogna, M.D., and Bucci, P. 1987. 'Aulin: a new modern drug in the treatment of inflammation in dentistry.' *Minerva Stomatologica* January-February *36*(1-2):101-3.

Bucci, E., Signoriello, G., Perrino, I.F., and Bucci, P. 1986. 'Clinico-pharmacological comparison between between enzyme-type anti-inflammatory agents postoperatively in oral surgery.' *Minerva Stomatologica* May *35*(5):503-6.

Dallas, P., Rekkas, D., and Choulis, N.H. 1989. 'HPLC determination of serratiopeptidase in biological fluids.' *Pharmazie* April *44*(4):297.

Esch, P.M., Gerngross, H., and Fabian, A. 1989. 'Reduction of postoperative swelling. Objective measurement of swelling of the upper ankle joint in treatment with serrapeptase— a prospective study.' *Fortschritte der Medizin 107*:67-8, 71-2.

Ijitsu, T., Yonezawa, K., and Ueno, M. 1986. 'Improved analysis of serrapeptase by high performance steric exclusion chromatography (SEC). I.' *Yakugaku Zasshi* January *106*(1):95-8.

Ishihara, Y., Kitamura, S., and Takaku, F. 1983. 'Experimental studies on distribution of cefotiam, a new beta-lactam antibiotic, in the lung and trachea of rabbits. II. Combined effects with serratiopeptidase.' *Japanese Journal of Antibiotics* October *36*(10):2665-70.

Kase, Y., Seo, H., Oyama, Y., Sakata, M., Tomoda, K., Takahama, K., Hitoshi, T., Okano, Y., and Miyata, T. 1982. 'A new method for evaluating mucolytic expectorant activity and its application. II. Application to two proteolytic enzymes, serratiopeptidase and seaprose.' *Arzneimittelforschung 32*:4 374-8.

Kee, W.H., Tan, S.L., Lee, V., and Salmon, Y.M. 1989. 'The treatment of breast engorgement with Serrapeptase (Danzen): a randomised double-blind controlled trial.' *Singapore Medical Journal* February *30*(1):48-54.

Koyama, A., Mori, J., Tokuda, H., Waku, M., Anno, H., Katayama, T., Murakami, K., Komatsu, H., Hirata, M., Arai, T., et al. 1986. 'Augmentation by serrapeptase of tissue permeation by cefotiam.' *Japanese Journal of Antibiotics* March *39*(3):761-71.

Kuettner, K., Sorgente, N., Croxen, R., Howell, D., and Pita, J. 1974. 'Lysozyme in Preosseous Cartilage. VII. Evidence for Physiological Role of Lysozyme in Normal Endochondral Calcificaion.' *Biochim Biophys Acta 372*:335.

Lee, H.S., Majima, Y., Sakakura, Y., and Kim, B.W. 1991. 'A technique for quantitative cytology of nasal secretions.' *European Archives of Otorhinolaryngology 248*(7):406-8.

Majima, Y., Hirata, K., Takeuchi, K., Hattori, M., and Sakakura, Y. 1990. 'Effects of orally administered drugs on dynamic viscoelasticity of human nasal mucus.' *American Review of Respiratory Disease* January *141*(1):79-83.

Majima, Y., Inagaki, M., Hirata, K., Takeuchi, K., Morishita, A., and Sakakura, Y. 1988. 'The effect of an orally administered proteolytic enzyme on the elasticity and viscosity of nasal mucus.' *Archives of Otorhinolaryngology 244*(6):355-9.

Malshe, P.C. 1998. 'Orally administered serratiopeptidase: can it work?' *Journal of the Association of Physicians of India* May *46*(5):492.

Malshe, P. C. 2000. 'A preliminary trial of serratiopeptidase in patients with carpal tunnel Syndrome.' *Journal of the Association of Physicians of India* November *48*(11):1130.

Mazzone, A., Catalani, M., Costanzo, M., Drusian, A., Mandoli, A., Russo, S., Guarini, E., and Vesperini, G. 1990. 'Evaluation of Serratia peptidase in acute or chronic inflammation of otorhinolaryngology pathology: a multicentre, double-blind, randomized trial versus placebo.' *Journal of International Medical Research 18*(5):379-88.

Merten, H.A., Muller, K., Drubel, F., and Halling, F. 1991. 'Volumetric verification of edema protection with Serrapeptase after third molar osteotomy.' *Deutsche Zeitschrift für Mund-, Kiefer- und Gesichts-Chirurgie 15*:302-5.

Miyata, K. 1980. 'Intestinal absorption of Serratia Peptidase.' *Journal of Applied Biochemistry 2*:111-16.

Moriya, N., Nakata, M., Nakamura, M., Takaoka, M., Iwasa, S., Kato, K., and Kakinuma, A. 1994. 'Intestinal absorption of serrapeptase (TSP) in rats.' *Biotechnology and Applied Biochemistry* 20(Pt 1):101-8.

Nakamura, S., Hashimoto, Y., Mikami, M., Yamanaka, E., Soma, T., Hino, M., Azuma, A., and Kudoh, S. 2003. 'Effect of the proteolytic enzyme serrapeptase in patients with chronic airway disease.' *Respirology* September 8(3):316-20.

Okumura, H., Watanabe, R., Kotoura, Y., Nakane, Y., and Tangiku, O. 1977. 'Effects of a proteolytic-enzyme preparation used concomitantly with an antibiotic in osteoarticular infections.' *Japanese Journal of Antibiotics* March 30(3):223-7.

Ovartlarnporn, B., Kulwichit, W., and Hiranniramol, S. 1991. 'Medication-induced esophageal injury: report of 17 cases with endoscopic documentation.' *American Journal of Gastroenterology* June 86(6):748-50.

Panagariya, A., and Sharma, A.K. 1999. 'A preliminary trial of serratiopeptidase in patients with carpal tunnel syndrome.' *Journal of the Association of Physicians of India* December 47(12):1170-2.

Salamone, P.R., and Wodzinski, R.J. 1997. 'Production, purification and characterization of a 50-kDa extracellular metalloprotease from *Serratia marcescens*.' *Applied Microbiology and Biotechnology* September 48(3):317-24.

Salvato, A., Zambruno, E., Ventrini, E., and Savio, G. 1984. 'Clinical experiments with a new oral anti-edema drug: nimesulide.' *Giornale di Stomatologia e di Ortognatodonzia* April-June 3(2):184-91.

Sasaki, S., Kawanami, R., Motizuki, Y., Nakahara, Y., Kawamura, T., Tanaka, A., and Watanabe, S. 2000. 'Serrapeptase-induced lung injury manifesting as acute eosiniphilic pneumonia.' *Nihon Kokyuki Gakkai Zasshi* July 38(7):540-4.

Scremin, S., Gini, M., Schiavi, M., Ciani, D., and Caprioglio, L. 1985. 'Comparison between imidazole-2-hydroxybenzoate and serratio-peptidase in the treatment of phlogistic diseases of the respiratory tract.' *Bollettino Chimico Farmaceutico* August 24(8):71S-75S.

Selan, L., Berlutti, F., Passariello, C., Comodi-Ballanti, M.R., and Thaller, M.C. 1993. 'Proteolytic enzymes: a new treatment strategy for prosthetic infections?' *Antimicrobial Agents and Chemotherapy* December 37(12):2618-21.

Shimizu, H., Ueda, M., Takai, T., Bito, T., Ichihashi, M., Muramatsu, T., and Shirai, T. 1999. 'A case of serratiopeptidase-induced subepidermal bullous dermatosis.' *British Journal of Dermatology* December 141(6):1139-40.

Shimura, S., Okubo, T., Maeda, S., Aoki, T., Tomioka, M., Shindo, Y., Takishima, T., and Umeya, K. 1983. 'Effect of expectorants on relaxation behavior of sputum viscoelasticity in vivo.' *Biorheology* 20(5):677-83.

Suzuki, K., Niho, T., Yamada, H., Yamaguchi, K., and Ohnishi, H. 1983. 'Experimental study of the effects of bromelain on the sputum consistency in rabbits.' *Nippon Yakurigaku Zasshi* March 81(3):211-6.

Tachibana, M., Mizukoshi, O., Harada, Y., Kawamoto, K., and Nakai, Y. 1984. 'A multi-centre, double-blind study of serrapeptase versus placebo in post-antrotomy buccal swelling.' *Pharmatherapeutica* 3(8):526-30.

Tanimoto, T., Fukuda, H., and Yamaha, T. 1986. 'Studies on the quality of enzyme preparations (VII)-serrapeptase preparation.' *Eisei Shikenjo Hokoku* (104):38-45.

Tanimoto, T., Fukuda, H., and Kawamura, J. 1983. 'On the quality of enzyme preparation (V) Serratiopeptidase preparation.' *Eisei Shikenjo Hokoku* (101):92-5.

Vicari, E., La Vignera, S., Battiato, C., and Arancio, A. 2005. 'Treatment with non-steroidal anti-inflammatory drugs in patients with amicrobial chronic prostato-vesiculitis: transrectal ultrasound and seminal findings.' *Minerva Urologica e Nefrologica* March 57(1):53-9.

Yamada, S., Ogawa, T., Nishimiya, J., Yuasa, T., and Taketazu, F. 2003. 'Masticator myopathy.' *Muscle and Nerve* July 28(1):123-7.

Yamazaki, F. 1967. *Pharmacol Japonica* 63:302-307.*

Yonkers, A.J. 1992. 'Sinusitis - Inspecting the causes and treatment.' Otolaryngology/Head/Neck Surg. Dept., Univ. of Nebraska Medical Center, United States Ear, Nose and Throat Journal 71/6:258-262.

Yoshida, K. 1983. 'Sfericase, a novel proteolytic enzyme.' *International Journal of Clinical Pharmacology, Therary, and Toxicology* September 21(9):439-46.

Research on enzymes and colon problems

Popiela, T., Kulig, J., Klek, S., Wachol, D., Bock, P. R., and Hanisch, J. 2000. 'Double-blind pilot-study on the efficacy of enzyme therapy in advanced colorectal cancer.' *Przegla'd Lekarski* 57(Suppl 5):142.

Popiela, T., Kulig, J., Hanisch, J., and Bock, P.R. 2001. 'Influence of a complementary treatment with oral enzymes on patients with colorectal cancers—an epidemiological retrolective cohort study.' *Cancer Chemotherapy and Pharmacology* July 47(Suppl):S55-63.

Ragnhammar, P., Hafstrom, L., Nygren, P., and Glimelius, B. 2001. 'A systematic overview of chemotherapy effects in colorectal cancer.' *Acta Oncologica* 40(2-3):282-308.

Other cancers

Beuth, J., Ost, B., Pakdaman, A., Rethfeldt, E., Bock, P.R., Hanisch, J., and Schneider, B. 2001. 'Impact of complementary oral enzyme application on the postoperative treatment results of breast cancer patients—results of an epidemiological multicentre retrolective cohort study.' *Cancer Chemotherapy and Pharmacology* July 47(Suppl):S45-54.

Gubareva, A.A. 1998. 'The use of enzymes in treating patients with malignant lymphoma with a large tumor mass.' *Likars'ka Sprava* August (6):141-3.

Hanul, V.L., Smolanka, I.I., and Ponomar'ova, O.V. 2000. 'Application of systemic enzyme therapy in combined treatment of patients with pulmonary cancer and malignant thymoma.' *Klinicheskaia Khirurgiia.* June (6):17-9.

Kaul, R., Mishra, B.K., Sutradar, P., Choudhary, V., and Gujral, M.S. 1999. 'The role of Wobe-Mugos in reducing acute sequele of radiation in head and neck cancers—a clinical phase-III randomized trial.' *Indian Journal of Cancer.* June-December 36(2-4):141-8.

Smolanka, I.I. 2000. 'Systemic enzyme therapy with the preparation Wobe-Mugos E in the combined treatment of lung cancer patients.' *Likars'ka Sprava* July-August (5):121-3.

Other research

Aldoori, W.H., Giovannucci, E.L., Rockett, H.R., Sampson, L., Rimm, E.B., and Willett, W.C. 1998. 'A prospective study of dietary fiber types and symptomatic diverticular disease in men.' *Journal of Nutrition 128*:714-9.

Bassetti, S., Frei, R., and Zimmerli, W. 1998. 'Fungemia with *Saccharomyces cerevisiae* after treatment with *Saccharomyces boulardii*'. *American Journal of Medicine 105:71-2.*

Bhounik, Y., Vahedi, K., Achour, L., Attar, A., Salfati, J., Pochart, P., Marteau, P., Flourie, B., Bornet, F., and Rambaud, J.C. 1999. 'Short-chain fructo-oligosaccharide administration dose-dependently increases fecal bifidobacteria in healthy humans.' *Journal of Nutrition 129*:113-6.

Bouhnik, Y., Flourie, B., D'Agay-Abensour, L., Pochart, P., Gramet, G., Durand, M., and Rambaud, J.C. 1997. 'Administration of transgalacto-oligosaccharides increases fecal bifidobacteria and modifies colonic fermentation metabolism in healthy humans.' *Journal of Nutrition 127*:444-8.

Brown, L., Rosner, B., Willett, W.W., and Sacks, F.M. 1999. 'Cholesterol-lowering effects of dietary fiber: a meta-analysis.' *American Journal of Clinical Nutrition 69*:30-42.

Chez, M. G., Buchanan, C.P., and Komen, J. 2002. 'L-Carnosine Therapy for Intractable Epilepsy in Childhood: Effect on EEG.' *Epilepsia 43*(7):65.

D'Souza, A.L., Rajkumar, C., Cooke, J., and Bulitt, C. 2002. 'Probiotics in prevention of antibiotic associated diarrhea: meta-analysis.' *British Medical Journal 324*:1361.

Heber, D., Yip, I., Ashley, J.M., Elashoff, D.A., Elashoff, R.M., and Go, V.L. 1999. 'Cholesterol-lowering effects of a proprietary Chinese red-yeast-rice dietary supplement.' *American Journal of Clinical Nutrition 69*:231-236.

Facchinetti, F., Nappi, R.E., Sances, M.G., Neri, I., Grandinetti, G., and Genazzani, A. 1997. 'Effects of a yeast-based dietary supplementation on premenstrual syndrome: A double-blind placebo-controlled study.' *Gynecologic and Obstetric Investigation 43*:120-124.

Fung, T.T., Hu, F.B., Pereira, M.A., Liu, S., Stampfer, M.J., Colditz, G.A., and Willett, W.C. 2002. 'Whole-grain intake and the risk of type 2 diabetes: a prospective study in men.' *American Journal of Clinical Nutrition 76*:535-40.

Antiviral/antimicrobial components in dairy

Liu, S., Willett, W.C., Stampfer, M.J., Hu, F.B., Franz, M., Sampson, L., Hennekens, C.H., and Manson, J.E. 2000. 'A prospective study of dietary glycemic load, carbohydrate intake, and risk of coronary heart disease in US women.' *American Journal of Clinical Nutrition 71*:1455-61.

Mansour-Ghanaei, F., Dehbasi, N., Yazdanparast, K., and Shafaghi, A. 2003. 'Efficacy of *S. boulardii* with antibiotics in acute amebiasis.' *World J Gastroenterology 9*:1832-1833.*

McKeown, N.M., Meigs, J.B., Liu, S., Saltzman, E., Wilson, P.W., and Jacques, P.F. 2004. 'Carbohydrate nutrition, insulin resistance, and the prevalence of the metabolic syndrome in the Framingham Offspring Cohort.' *Diabetes Care* 27:538-46.

McKeown, N.M., Meigs, J.B., Liu, S., Wilson, P.W., and Jacques, P.F. 2002. 'Whole-grain intake is favorably associated with metabolic risk factors for type 2 diabetes and cardiovascular disease in the Framingham Offspring Study.' *American Journal of Clinical Nutrition* 76:390-8.

Olson, R.E. Vitamin K. In: Shils, M., Olson, J.A., Shike, M., and Ross, A.C. editors 1999. *Nutrition in Health and Disease* 9th edition. Baltimore, Maryland. Williams & Wilkins.

Pereira, M.A, O'Reilly, E., Augustsson, K., Fraser, G.E., Goldbourt, U., Heitmann, B.L., Hallmans, G., Knekt, P., Liu, S., Pietinen, P., Speigelman, D., Stevens, J., Virtamo, J., Willett, W.C., and Ascheria, A. 2004. 'Dietary fiber and risk of coronary heart disease: a pooled analysis of cohort studies.' *Archives of Internal Medicine* 164:370-6.

Rimm, E.B., Ascherio, A., Giovannucci, E., Spiegelman, D., Stampfer, M.J., and Willett, W.C. 1996. 'Vegetable, fruit, and cereal fiber intake and risk of coronary heart disease among men.' *Journal of the American Medical Association* 275:447-51.

Roberfroid, M. 1993. 'Dietary fibre, inulin and oligofructose. A review comparing their physiological effects.' *Critical Reviews in Food Science and Nutrition* 33:103-48.

Roberfroid, M.B., Van Loo, J.A., and Gibson, G.R. 1998. 'The bifidogenic nature of chicory inulin and its hydrolysis products.' *Journal of Nutrition* 128:11-9.

Schellenberg, D., Bonington, A., Champion, C.M., Lancaster, R., and Main, J. 1994. 'Treatment of *C. difficile* diarrhea with Brewer's yeast.' *Lancet* 343:171-172.

Schulze, M.B., Liu, S., Rimm, E.B., Manson, J.E., Willett, W.C., and Hu, F.B. 2004. 'Glycemic index, glycemic load, and dietary fiber intake and incidence of type 2 diabetes in younger and middle-aged women.' *American Journal of Clinical Nutrition* 80:348-56.

Surawicz, C.M., McFarland, L.V., Greenberg, R.N., et al. 2000. 'The search for a better treatment for recurrent *C. difficile* disease: use of high-dose vancomycin combined with *S. boulardii*.' *Clinical Infectious Diseases* 31:1012-1017.

Van Dokkum, W., Wezendonk, B., Srikumar, T.S., and Van den Heuvel, E.G. 1999. 'Effect of nondigestible oligosaccharides on large-bowel functions, blood lipid concentrations and glucose absorption in young healthy male subjects.' *European Journal of Clinical Nutrition* 53:1-7.

Van Horn, L. 1997. 'Fiber, lipids, and coronary heart disease. A statement for healthcare professionals from the Nutrition Committee, American Heart Association.' *Circulation* 95:2701-4.

Index

Disclaimer

The information contained herein is not intended to diagnose, treat, prevent, or cure any disease, or to provide specific medical advice. Its intention is solely to inform and to educate. If you have any questions about the relationship between nutrition, supplements, and your health, seek the advice of a qualified health practitioner. The reader and associated health professionals are responsible for evaluating the risks of any therapy reviewed in this book. Those responsible made every effort possible to thoroughly research the accuracy of the information and assume no responsibility for errors, inaccuracies, or omissions. Digestive enzymes are an unregulated dietary supplement classified as a safe food by the Food and Drug Administration in the United States. Opinions and experiences contained herein do not reflect the position of any enzyme manufacturer, formulator, or distributor. The author has no financial interests with any enzyme or supplement manufacturer or distributor. The organizations and companies mentioned herein do not specifically endorse any particular therapy or product.

All product and company names are the properties of the
respective organizations.